Podiatric Medicine and Surgery
A Monograph series

Edited by

Morton D. Fielding, D.P.M.

Volume I : Surgical Treatment of Hallux-Abducto Valgus
Volume II : Surgical Treatment of the Intractable Plantar Keratoma
Volume III : Skin Tumors of the Foot: Diagnosis and Treatment

Skin Tumors of the Foot: Diagnosis and Treatment

Edited by

Morton D. Fielding, D.P.M.
Consulting Podiatrist to the National Institute of Health

Contributors

Steven J. Berlin, D.P.M., Chairman
and Members of Maryland Podiatric
Residency Research Committee.

FUTURA
PUBLISHING COMPANY
1974

Published by
Futura Publishing Company, Inc.
295 Main Street
Mount Kisco, New York 10549

L.C.: 74-82020
ISBN: 0-87993-043-8

Printed in the U.S.A.

This book is dedicated to our wives
and
to the future of podiatry, research, and education.

Contributors

Steven J. Berlin, D.P.M., F.A.C.F.S.
Director Podiatry Research, Maryland Podiatric Residency Program; Assistant Director of Podiatric Surgery, Maryland Podiatric Residency Program; Chairman, Tissue Committee, American College of Foot Surgeons; Special Consultant in Oncology, Journal American Podiatry Association; Chief of Podiatry Service, Spring Grove Hospital Center; Podiatry Consultant, Rosewood and Mt. Wilson Hospital Center, and Fort Howard V.A. Hospital.

Steven A. Brownstein, D.P.M.
Podiatry Staff, Crownsville State Hospital Center.

Robert W. Geister, D.P.M.
Podiatry Staff, Rosewood Hospital Center.

Gary Gordon, D.P.M.
Podiatry Staff, Mt. Wilson Hospital Center.

Larry S. Hotchkiss, D.P.M.
Podiatry Staff, Springfield Hospital Center.

Frank L. Levy, D.P.M.
Podiatry Staff, Rosewood Hospital Center

Richard C. Stewart, D.P.M.
Podiatry Staff, Spring Grove Hospital Center.

Special Consultants

Ronald Goldner, M.D.
Diplomate American Board of Dermatology; Assistant Professor of Dermatology, University of Maryland Hospital; Chief of Dermatology, Maryland General Hospital, Baltimore. Md.

William V. R. Shellow, M.D.
Diplomate American Board of Dermatology; Clinical Assistant Professor of Dermatology, University of California, Los Angeles, California; Assistant Chief of Dermatology, V.A. Wadsworth Hospital Center, Los Angeles, California.

Isidore Zeligman, M.D.
Diplomate American Board of Dermatology; Associate Professor of Dermatology, John Hopkins University School of Medicine, Baltimore, Maryland; Chief of Dermatology, Sinai Hospital, Baltimore, Maryland.

Special Acknowledgment

Today's understanding of a specific topic has become so complex in our society that no specialized book is written entirely without other opinions, teachings, and philosophies.

Our committee is deeply indebted to our medical colleagues, Drs. Ronald Goldner, William V. R. Shellow, and Isidore Zeligman for their enthusiastic assistance in the preparation of this text.

This book owes sincerest thanks to the special individuals who labored so efficiently in its preparation: Mrs. Eva Plude, Mrs. Carolyn Lynch, Mrs. Eileen Berlin and Mrs. Marcene Michaelson our secretaries.

We also wish to thank all members of the Maryland Podiatric Residency Research Committee and particularly Drs. Irvin Donick, Lawrence Block, Anthony Costa, Lanny Rubin, Harvey Brown, Michael Feinstein, Neil Sheffler, Paul Sheitel, and Bruce Lebowitz for their support and guidance in the program.

Preface

There is a great tendency today toward provincialism among the many branches of medicine. Within the various specialties and sub-specialties, this attitude is even more pronounced. We all feel proficient within our chosen disciplines, but it is uncommon to look beyond our own immediate purviews.

All of medicine is becoming focused upon an important goal; that of continuing education. Pressures to keep abreast of current thinking originally came from without, but now are coming increasingly from within, for we all realize that not keeping up is to fail those who rely upon our skills. What we once mastered while in graduate school, post-graduate training, and what we improve upon in continued specialty practice must be constantly supplemented by journals, seminars, local and national meetings, and by up-to-date texts such as this one written by Dr. Steven J. Berlin, et al.

Dr. Berlin and his associates have given us a monograph dealing with skin tumors of the foot — but since none of our specialties exist within a void, they have overlapped such fields as pathology, dermatology, oncology, epidemiology, and virology. They have used the sometimes fortuitous occurrence of a lesion on the skin of the foot as a springboard for a comprehensive discussion of their subject, be it melanoma, pyogenic granuloma, squamous cell carcinoma or verruca.

The individual sections are presented with clarity, and they should prove as useful to experienced practioners seeking an up-to-date topic review — as to students perusing a subject for the first time.

The podiatry research committee's scholarship and devoted effort are evident in their extensive sectional bibliographies. This monograph will prove to be a valuable reference work in the library of anyone interested in the skin, whether their degree is D.P.M. or M.D.

Having read this work, it became more apparent than ever that our disciplines closely interact, and that which interests one of us will usually interest the other. More importantly, the needs of all of our patients will better be served by sharing our collective knowledge.

If this book can expand the outlook of each of us within our own specialty — as I fully expect it will — then Dr. Berlin has fully and commendably completed the task which he has set for himself and his committee.

William Van Ronkel Shellow, M.D.

Clinical Assistant Professor of Medicine/Dermatology University of California at Los Angeles; and Assistant Chief of Dermatology Veterans Administration Wadsworth Hospital Center Los Angeles, California

Table of Contents

Contributors vii
Preface xi

Section I — **Skin Tumors of the Foot** by: Steven J. Berlin, D.P.M., F.A.C.F.S.
- Introduction 3
- Diagnosis 5
- Treatment 11

Section II — **Viral Type Growths Involving the Pedal Skin** by: Steven J. Berlin, D.P.M., F.A.C.F.S., and Richard Stewart, D.P.M.
- Introduction 17
- Verruca Plantaris 18
- Molluscum Contagiosum 47
- Herpes Simplex 50
- Herpes Zoster 52

Section III — **Hyperkeratotic Lesions and Related Skin Growths** by: Steven J. Berlin, D.P.M., F.A.C.F.S., and Frank L. Levy, D.P.M.
- Introduction 63
- Idiopathic Hereditary Keratosis
  1. Keratosis Palmaris et Plantaris Hereditaris (Unna Thost) 68
  2. Keratosis Punctata 68
  3. Keratosis Striata 75
  4. Mal de Meleda 76
  5. Papillon-LeFevre Syndrome .. 77
- Precancerous Keratosis
  1. Arsenical Keratosis 79

2. Occupational Keratosis 81
3. Actinic Keratosis 82
4. Cutaneous Horn 84
5. Keratoacanthoma 87
Cutaneous Lesions and Manifestations of Systemic Disease
1. Acanthosis Nigricans 90
2. Arthritic Diseases 92
3. Bullous Pemphigoid 96
4. Diabetes Mellitus 97
5. Erythema Elevatum Diutinum 100
6. Mastocytosis Syndrome 103
7. Mycobacterial Infections 104
8. Mycosis Fungoides 104
9. Papulo Squamous Diseases ... 107
10. Parasitic Infections 108
11. Reiter's Syndrome 110
12. Syphilis 111

Section IV **Nevi and Malignant Skin Lesions of the Foot** by: Steven J. Berlin, D.P.M., F.A.C.F.S., Larry S. Hotchkiss, D.P.M., and Steven A. Brownstein, D.P.M.
Nevi 119
Melanoma 125
Basal Cell Carcinoma 144
Squamous Cell Carcinoma 155
Bowen's Disease 165

Section V **Tumors of the Pedal Skin and Related Connective Tissue Neoplasms** by: Steven J. Berlin, D.P.M., F.A.C.F.S., Gary Gordon, D.P.M., and Robert W. Geister, D.P.M.
Adnexal Tumors
1. Eccrine Poroma 181
2. Porokeratosis Plantaris Discreta 184

3. Sebaceous "Pilar" Cyst 187
4. Epidermal Inclusion Cyst 188
Fibrous Tumors
1. Fibroma 195
2. Periungual Fibroma 196
3. Recurrent Digital Fibroma of Childhood 200
4. Dermatofibroma 201
5. Keloids & Hypertrophic Scars 205
6. Cutaneous Mucous Cysts (Myxoid Cysts) 219
7. Dermatofibrosarcoma Protuberans 221
Hemangioma
1. Strawberry 224
2. Spider Nevus 224
3. Port-Wine Stain 224

SECTION I

SKIN TUMORS OF THE FOOT

Introduction

It has often been said that tumors of the foot are very rare; however, it is just the contrary. Malignancies are uncommon; benign tumors of the foot are an everyday common occurrence, but many times are overlooked or misdiagnosed. The common plantar wart is the most frequent lesion that will be seen presenting various forms of symptoms in the daily practice of the podiatrist. As common as warts may be, they too are very often misdiagnosed.

Tumors of the foot are certainly not a new occurrence and they have been described in the literature before Christ. The pedal skin may only represent approximately 2% of the total skin surface of the body, yet it is the author's opinion that more than 2% of the neoplasms found on the human body are located on the foot. In our personal experience hundreds of lesions are removed yearly in daily practice.

Many of these lesions affecting the foot are seldom reported by the clinician. The foot is the most abused portion of the body, and the most neglected, and is easily hidden by shoes and socks. Perhaps for these reasons, neoplasms of not only the pedal skin, but also other areas of the foot have only been recorded on sporadic occasions.

The purpose of this monograph is to assist the podiatrist and other clinicians in the clinical diagnosis and management of skin tumors as they affect the foot.

The skin is the largest organ system in the human body and like most other organs, once permanently damaged, cannot be replaced. The skin consists of two main portions: the epidermis and the dermis. It has three kinds of exocrine glands, but does not have any endocrine glands. The sole or plantar surface of the foot has special characteristics in relation to its thickness and functions which differ from all other areas of the skin, except perhaps for that of the palms.

The epidermis consists of five layers and is ectodermal in origin. The deepest layer of the epidermis is known as the basal layer, or stratum germinativum, which lies just above the connective tissue layers of the foot. It is within this layer that the greatest amount of regenerative power exists. The stratum spinosum, or prickle cell layer, is the second layer and comprises most of the epidermis. It plays an important part in the nutritional and metabolic exchanges of the cells. The stratum granulosum, the third layer of the plantar skin, usually consists of two to five rows of cells. It is possible that this layer of the epidermis may have a specific role in the process of keratinization. The stratum lucidum is the fourth layer and is more prominent on the plantar epidermis. The outer layer of the epidermis is known as the stratum corneum or horny layer. It is this layer that is constantly being replaced by the epidermis in order to provide protection for the skin. The color of the skin is usually determined by the melanin pigment which may be present in the basal layers of the epidermis and the vascular status of the dermis.

The dermis, or underlying connective tissue structures, are derived from the mesoderm. It is within these structures that the epidermis derives its nutrients and tactile senses. The dermis or corium support the epidermis and separate it from the subcutaneous fatty tissue. The dermis is divided into two sections, the papillary and the reticular layers. In many instances, tumors affecting the epidermis also affect the dermal layers of the skin and vice versa.

The skin serves many functions for the human body:

1) Protection — The epidermis protects the body against various forms of mechanical insults or noxious substances.
2) Transportation — A complex organization of blood and lymphatic vessels exists.
3) Secretion — The human skin may act as an exocrine gland.
4) Excretion — Excretion of various waste such as urea, sweat, and carbon dioxide through the epithelial skin.
6) Sensory reception — Certain specialized epithelial cells may help serve as an intermediary for various nervous transmissions.
7) Reproduction — Specific cells of the epithelium have a tendency to perpetuate one another. Skin tumors of the foot can affect any one of the various epithelial layers or may affect all the epithelial layers and certain underlying structures, depending on the specific type of neoplasms.

Diagnosis

The most important aspect of diagnosis is recognizing that an abnormal growth is definitely taking place. One must possess the knowledge or ability to classify the various structural changes which are taking place when observing a definite change in the skin.

There may be many skin manifestations of disease which can easily be confused with that of a skin tumor. The most common of these manifestations may be by macules, papules, vesicles, bullae, pustules, as well as various forms of hyperkeratosis. The history obtained from the individual patient may be the primary clue in one's diagnosis of various growths on the pedal skin. Since there are so many types of dermatitis or other skin lesions which closely resemble neoplasms, and since so many skin lesions have the tendency to mimic one another, it is essential to obtain a laboratory diagnosis, such as a biopsy, to confirm one's clinical opinion. It is our opinion that pathological diagnosis is a must in today's medico-legal society.

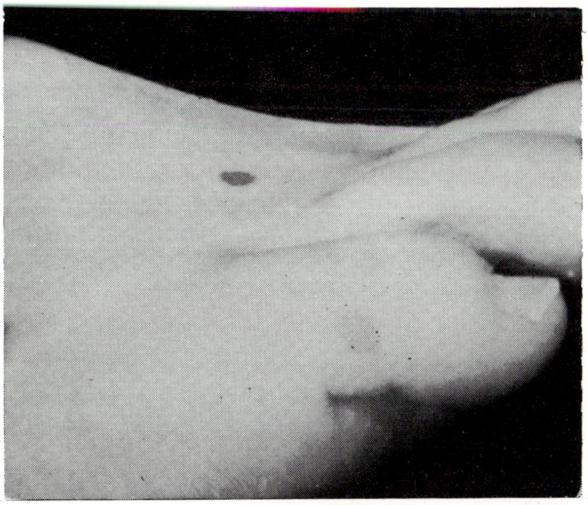

FIGURE 1-1

Two of most common lesions found on the foot are the common mole, dorsum of the foot and the verruca, fifth toe.

Skin lesions of the foot may take on various shapes and sizes. Skin tumors on the dorsal surfaces of the foot very frequently differ from the same tumor when it is located on the plantar surface. This differentiation is probably due to weight bearing pressures on the plantar surface. Skin tumors on the sole of the foot are often more deeply seated within the epidermis and are often accompanied by hyperkeratotic changes. Unfortunately, people have different ways of describing the gross anatomy of tumors, which often leads to much confusion in one's diagnosis. Yet, diagnosis of various tumors affecting the pedal skin may be classified as 1) lesions which may be flat in relation to the skin plane, such as macules, 2) lesions which may be elevated above the skin plane, such as nodules or cysts, pustules, and plaques, or 3) lesions which are depressed or below the skin plane, such as scars or ulcers, excoriations, and even atrophy of the lesion itself.

Probably the most important aspect of clinical diagnosis is that of the change or sudden change in the appearance of any skin

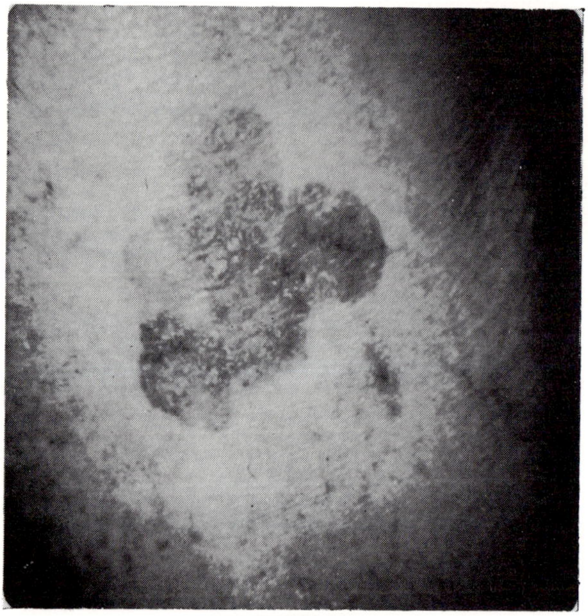

FIGURE 1-2

Bowen's Lesion on lower leg revealing a well defined lesion.

lesion. A noticeable differentiation in any skin lesion may not only help in one's diagnosis, but may also help in determining one's treatment.

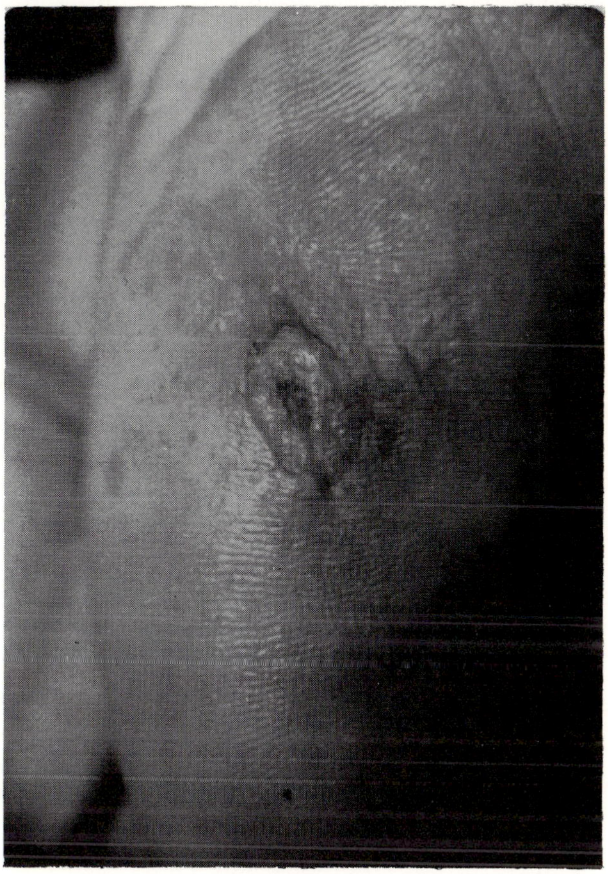

FIGURE 1-3

Bowen's Lesion on sole. These lesions are more difficult to clinically diagnose. (Courtesy Richard Gibbs, M.D., New York City)

LABORATORY DIAGNOSIS

The most important laboratory diagnosis in assisting the podiatrist in his clinical judgement is that of a biopsy. Punch biopsy is a very easy surgical procedure to obtain an accurate pathological diagnosis. Different size punch biopsies are available. The most important area for a biopsy is not the central portion of the lesion itself, but a portion of the lesion and surrounding normal tissue. In obtaining both normal and abnormal tissue, the histological differentiation makes a more complete microscopic picture.

Evaluation of the blood and urine of the individual is most often of very little value in assisting in one's diagnosis of skin tumors of the foot. However, certain pathological lesions which are present on the pedal skin may be due to underlying systemic disease, such as diabetes, tuberous sclerosis, Von Recklinghausen's Disease, hypercholesterolemia and even syphilis. Certain vascular lesions which manifest themselves on the foot may be studied by laboratory tests using direct smears which can be stained with Wright's stain. Other cutaneous lesions, such as those of syphilis, may be confirmed by immediate darkfield examination. A scraping (KOH examination) and culture for fungi can also be of great assistance.

DIFFERENTIAL DIAGNOSIS

One of the most important aspects of differential diagnosis is the patient's history. When questioning an individual patient, it is extremely important to obtain a family history and not just the history of the present illness. There are certain characteristic diseases, such as Von Recklinghausen's Disease or tuberous sclerosis, as well as many hyperkeratotic lesions, which may be hereditary in nature. The color of a lesion may also give a clue to one's diagnosis. Hyperkeratosis, for instance, appears as a whitish type of lesion. Various types of skin fibromas may have a brownish color or appearance. The location of lesions may also present a definite clue to differential diagnosis. Certain lesions may have a predilection for hairy skin areas of the pedal foot, such as sebaceous or "pilar" cysts, whereas, epidermal inclusion cysts are more commonly located on the plantar surfaces of the foot. Lesions, whether above or below the skin, may also assist in one's clinical differential diagnosis.

Knowing and understanding the descriptive terminology of skin lesions can also help one's clinical judgement. Some of the more important descriptive lesions are as follows:

1) *Macules* — A macule may be a flat lesion representing only a color change in relation to the skin surface. It is usually a circumscribed lesion and may vary in size. They may be pigmented or non-pigmented. An example may be a junctional nevus. Macules may also give clues to various systemic diseases, such as tuberous sclerosis, and perhaps certain forms of leprosy.

2) *Papules* — A papule is an elevated lesion, usually solid in nature, with the majority of the lesion being elevated above the skin plane. Papules may vary in color, such as a violaceous hue type which is seen in lichen planus. There also may be rounded types of papules as seen in molluscum contagiosum.

3) *Plaques* — Plaques are usually large elevations which often cover a large area of the skin. However, plaques are often a coalescence of papules, such as those seen in mycosis fungoides or psoriasis. Various forms of yellcwish like plaques may be seen in lesions associated with diabetes mellitus, such as necrobiosis, lipoidica diabeticorum.

4) *Nodules* — Nodules are usually solid, palpable lesions which often extend into the dermis, or even into the subcutaneous tissues. Various nodules may develop as a result of benign skin changes, but also those of malignant degeneration. The various examples of nodules may be those of verrucae vulgaris, basal cell carcinoma and even keratoacanthoma.

5) *Vesicles and Bullae* — These are usually elevated skin lesions and often contain fluid. Vesicles and bullae may arise from various levels of skin cleavage, either being involved in the epidermis, or at the epidermal-dermal junctions. Various forms of vesicles and bullae which may present themselves on the foot may be those of herpes zoster, herpes simplex or other systemic diseases such as bullous pemphigoid.

6) *Pustules* — Pustules are usually circumscribed, raised skin lesions that often contain a purulent material. An example of pustule on the pedal skin may be that of impetigo or pustular psoriasis. Again, herpes simplex or herpes zoster may also present themselves with pustules.

7) *Cysts* — Cysts usually present themselves as sac type lesions containing liquid or semi-solid material. The most common of these cysts are known as epidermal or keratin cysts. The epidermal cysts have become more frequently seen in the foot, perhaps due to the barefoot generation which is now taking place in this country.

8) *Atrophy* — Epidermal atrophy is usually recognized by a thinning or transparent type of epidermis usually associated with a loss of epidermal cells. An example of atrophy may be an ulcer.

9) *Sclerosis* — Sclerotic lesions may present themselves as diffuse, hard, or indurated skin areas which are often circumscribed in nature. These lesions are usually detected more on palpation of the foot. A good example of sclerosis is scleroderma. Keloids may also be a form of sclerosis.

10) *Excoriations* — Excoriations are usually seen in pruritic lesions, which may present themselves as excavations of the epidermis or as linear or punctate losses of the epidermis. It can be a scratch mark.

11) *Fissures* — Fissures usually appear as linear cleavages in the skin, and are often seen in various forms of dermatosis involving the foot.

12) *Ulcers* — Ulcers are usually destructive type lesions where there has been destruction of both the epidermis and the dermal layers of the skin and even the underlying subcutaneous tissue. The causes of ulcers are numerous; however, its location and general appearance may help in one's diagnosis of the etiology.

Treatment

Treatment of skin tumors of the foot is probably the easiest aspect in caring for the individual patient. A substantial treatment can only be performed after an adequate diagnosis of the involved neoplasm has been made, and an understanding of that specific lesion has been evaluated. Once an adequate diagnosis and understanding of the present problem is made, a specific form of treatment may be instituted, which will hopefully result in a cure.

There are numerous forms of therapy one can institute in the treatment of skin lesions affecting the foot. Unfortunately, the simplest form of therapy is not always the best mode of treatment. Even the most radical forms of therapy often do not always result in a cure.

CHEMOTHERAPY

Chemotherapy is probably the simplest and most common form of therapy instituted by podiatrists. There are numerous forms of chemicals that one may employ, whether they be keratolytic types of drugs, or various blistering agents. These chemicals, however, when applied to the skin, should only be applied in subdestructive doses since a lethal dose to the skin may produce severe scarring and other unnecessary complications. The greatest advantage, however, of various forms of chemicals used in the treatment of topical skin tumors is that the clinician has the ability to use certain prescribed amounts or concentrations of the chemical being employed.

CRYOTHERAPY

Cryotherapy is another means of applying specific agents which will help create destruction of the specific lesion involved. The advantages of both chemical and freezing agents are that often they leave little or no scarring.

ELECTROCAUTERY

Electrocautery is a very popular form of treatment in various skin lesions, and is perhaps best utilized where there are multiple lesions. This prevents various surgical excisions of multiple lesions, and reduces the scarring and cosmetic effects which surgery may leave. Unfortunately, electrocautery also has its dangers such as over-destruction or over-utilization by burning through normal tissue, creating perhaps greater scars.

RADIATION THERAPY

Radiation therapy may be utilized in some of the more resistant type tumors. Unfortunately, it takes very skilled individuals to employ it. Over-utilization of X-rays may create severe scarring and further destructive lesions which may be a greater hazard than the original lesion. Radiation therapy on the foot may create even greater disadvantages because of the very bony surfaces which are present in the foot. Therefore radiation therapy, in regards to foot lesions, should only be utilized when absolutely necessary.

SURGERY

Surgical excision of the skin tumor of the foot is probably the easiest and most successful form of eradication of growths. Unfortunately, certain lesions may be of such size that adequate excision and normal skin closure may not be possible. If such a situation does arise, skin grafting can be utilized to cover the defect. Skin grafting in the foot, however, may not be as successful as on other areas of the body, particularly on the plantar surfaces of the foot where the skin is so specialized that donor tissue may not be adequate to support the defect.

PROGNOSIS

Fortunately most tumors of the foot are benign lesions and simple excision or other modes of therapy are usually quite successful. Malignancies of the skin, however, do create great hazards, and may cause death if inadequate treatment is performed. Early recognition of both benign and malignant skin tumors of the foot by the podiatrist or the clinician is imperative for an excellent prognosis.

BIBLIOGRAPHY

Cade, S.: Soft tissue tumors: Their natural history and treatment. *Royal Society of Medicine Proceedings,* **44**:19-36, 1951.
Conway, H. et al: *Surgery of Tumors of the Skin,* 2nd edition. Charles C. Thomas Publishers, Springfield, Illinois, 1966.
Costello, M. and Gibbs, R. C.: *The Palms and Soles in Medicine.* Charles C. Thomas Publishers, Springfield, Illinois, 1967.
Dorlands, I.: *Medical Dictionary,* 23rd edition. W. B. Saunders Company, Philadelphia, 1960.
Fitzpatrick, et al: *Dermatology in General Medicine.* McGraw-Hill, Inc., 1971.
Lever, W. F.: *Histopathology of the Skin,* 4th edition. J. B. Lippincott, Philadelphia, 1967.
Montgomery, R. M.: Painful cutaneous lesions of the feet. *Southern Medical Journal,* **63**:615-619, 1970.
Rook, A. et al: *Textbook of Dermatology.* Davis, Philadelphia, 1968.
Roy, S. L.: Simple tumors, cysts, and some minor surgical conditions. *Indian Medical Journal,* **60**:253-256, 1966.
Samitz, M. H. and Dana, A. S.: *Cutaneous Lesions of the Lower Extremities.* J. B. Lippincott, Philadelphia, 1971.
Weinstein, F. (Editor): *Principles and Practice of Podiatry.* Lea and Febiger, Philadelphia, 1968.
Yale, I.: *Podiatric Medicine.* The Williams and Wilkins Company, Baltimore, Maryland, 1974.

SECTION II

VIRAL TYPE GROWTHS INVOLVING THE PEDAL SKIN

Introduction

By definition, a tumor is a mass of new tissue which usually persists and grows independently of its surrounding structures, and which has no physiologic use.[48] A papilloma is an epithelial tumor in which the cells cover finger-like processes or ridges of stroma (dermis). Included in the category papilloma are:

1. The verrucae (vulgaris, plana, filiform, plantaris, mosaic) and condyloma acuminata.
2. A group which includes nevus verrocosus, senile keratosis, seborrheic keratosis, cutaneous horns, and acanthosis nigricans.[146]

The first group of papillomas are caused by infection with a particular epidermotropic virus. There is good evidence that the papova virus causes all of these verrucous papillomas.[7,112] The clinical and histologic differences are due to the type of skin and environment where the tumor is found. The majority of the discussion of verrucae will be directed toward the most common variety on the foot, verruca plantaris, most of it is applicable to verruca vulgaris and mosaic verruca.

The general use of the electron microscope in the early 1950's made the study of viral diseases a much more exact science. Noyes reviewed the methods of electron microscopy and gave an excellent description of the structure of the human wart virus in 1951.[119] It is one of a group called papova viruses (papova being an acronym from papilloma [pa], polyoma [po], and vacuolating [va] due to their similarity to the Shope virus which causes rabbit papillomas. The human papova virus (HPV) group (14) is shaped like an icosohedron with a diameter of 530 angstroms (making it a medium-sized virus) and containing 72 capsomeres.[60] The virus particle consists of an outer shell of protein (capsomeres) and an inner core of DNA. It is this DNA which replicates and multiplies in the nuclei of epidermal cells causing them to grow in an abnormal fashion.

Not all viral skin tumors found on the foot are papillomatous. Molluscum contagiosum is a nodular disease caused by a different epidermotropic virus.

Verruca Plantaris

Warts were, until recent advances in medical technology, usually associated with clandestine properties as a result of their refractoriness to therapy, recurrence, and tendency to spontaneously disappear. Mark Twain's colorful account of Tom Sawyer's favorite cure for warts illustrates this fact quite well: "You got to go all by yourself to the middle of the woods, when you know there's a spunk-water stump, and just as it's midnight you back up against the stump and jam your hand in and say: 'Barley corn, barley corn, injum meal shorts, spunk-water, spunk-water, swaller these warts,' then walk away quick, eleven steps, with your eyes shut, and then turn around three times and walk home without speaking to anybody. Because if you speak, the charm's busted."[164]

Incidence

The peak incidence of plantar warts is in children from age 7 to 15, and the incidence decreases in a linear manner with increasing age.[76] Most epidemiologic studies of verruca plantaris have been conducted on school populations. In these studies the incidence ranged from less than 1% to as high as 6.8%.[2,36,70,165,]

Etiology

Many early investigators believed warts were caused by some cellular organism, probably a bacteria, because they could transmit the warts to other subjects using an unfiltered wart extract.[90] Ciuffo first suspected a virus as the etiology of warts in 1907 when he reported the development of warts on one of his own fingers at the site of innoculation of a sterile, cell-free filtrate of verrucae homologous tissue.[37] Subsequent studies supported Ciuffo's suggestion that a virus was the transmissible agent. In 1951, Lyell and Miles presented a study of the eosinophilic inclusion bodies which could be demonstrated in the cytoplasm and nucleus of cells from myrmecia (plantar verrucae); this study further supported the theory that verrucae were caused by a

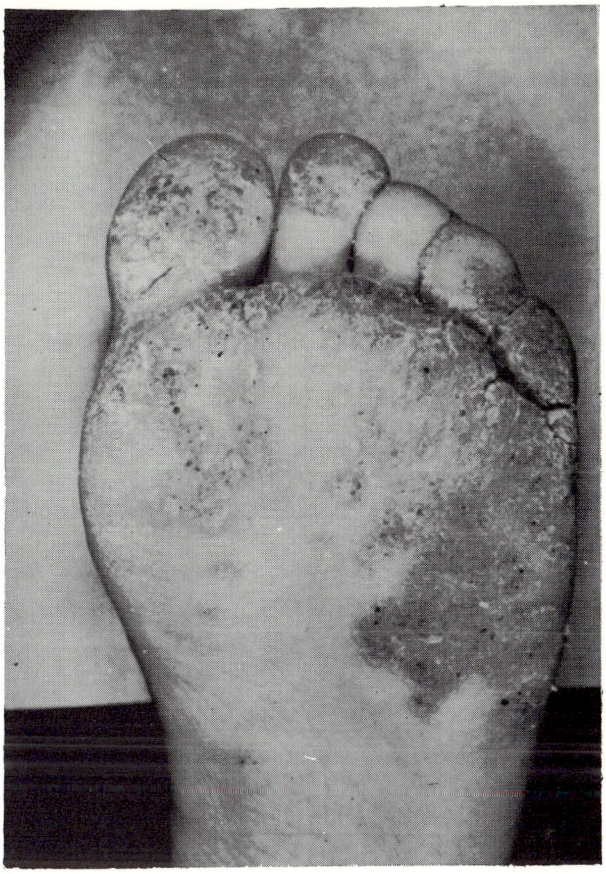

FIGURE 2-1

Mosaic Verruca: Severe and difficult lesions to treat. May or may not be painful on weight bearing. (Courtesy Ronald Goldner, M.D., Baltimore, Maryland)

filterable virus.[98] Almeida and associates discovered basophilic inclusion bodies in both common and plantar warts, which they believed suggest viral multiplication.[7]

Pathogenesis

Several studies offer good evidence that warts are indeed transmitted from one individual to another, usually by indirect contact. The most common forms of indirect contact occur in communal bathing areas, recreational areas, and school physical education areas.[36,70,104,149] The presence of excessive moisture and inadequate cleaning in these areas also appears to be related to a higher incidence.[70] It is difficult to assess the susceptibility of particular populations, ages, or sexes, because experimental innoculation of wart extracts to new hosts have been less than successful.[60 101]

However, homologous auto-innoculation has been successful experimentally, and is probably quite common clinically.[37,64] Massing and Epstein reported that new warts formed three times as often in children with present or previous verrucae.[103] Apparently most hosts can only support a limited number of colonies of the papova virus, usually one to three warts.[70] Mendelson and Klignan cultured myrmecia (plantar verrucae) and auto-innoculated extracts into the same subjects producing banal (common) warts in about 50%.[112]

The incubation period for the human papova virus is quite variable; it may range from one to 21 months, the average being four months.[103] There is evidence that the virus can live as a member of the normal cutaneous flora of the stratum spinosum for long periods of time.[64] In fact, some families of school children with plantar warts were found to have the wart virus present in the flora of their skin.[70] This may account for the wide variance in time lapse regarding recurrences and growths of new colonies following treatment of previous verrucae.

Most verrucae plantaris are found in weight-bearing areas (86%-87% in one study)[70] such as the ball and heel of the foot, similarly, most quiescent, non-clinical colonies of wart viruses are found in pressure areas.[101] Thus, most authors believe trauma plays a part in the successful innoculation of verrucae into the skin.[11,139] The excessive pressure and friction in the feet of athletes and patients with structural foot deformities may account for the high incidence of verruca plantaris in these groups. Also, hyperhidrosis apparently is related to the presence of verrucae.[139]

No specific anti-viral therapy has been developed. The infected patient must depend on his own immunologic defense system to combat the causative virus. This immunologic response is of two types: the humoral, or circulating antibody-type immunity, which is well documented; and the cell-mediated, or

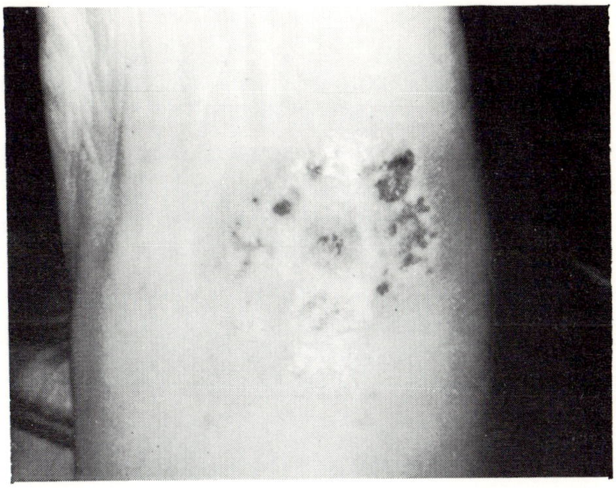

FIGURE 2-2

Plantar Verruca: Multiple plantar lesions of the heel undergoing self-destruction. Often these lesions become hemmorrhagic in color and painful.

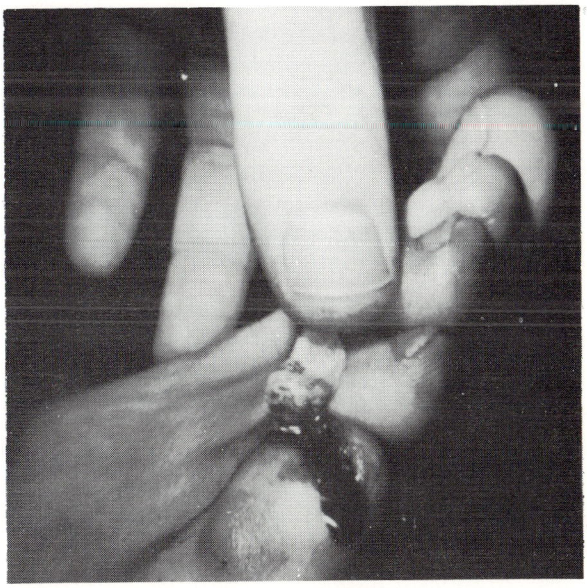

FIGURE 2-3

Subungual Verruca: Verruca underlying the nail is often misleading in diagnosis. Removal of nail must be performed prior to therapy.

lymphocyte-type immunity, which is presently being studied. As verrucae are a viral disease of the skin, it follows that the body must form an antibody response to the antigenic stimulus (the virus). In 1965 Almeida and Goffe found demonstratable antibodies inside wart tissue, and also circulating in the sera in 45% of their subjects.[6] They believed the lack of antibodies in the remaining patients was because "the wart virus is restricted to the upper layers of epidermis which has poor contact with the humoral system and therefore, little opportunity for stimulating antibody." In 1965, Walter and associates discovered a specific antigen in verrucous tissue which was detectible with flourescent-tagged antibody.[168] The antibodies were found to be of the IgG type.

Bunny states in 1971 that the IgG antibodies were not responsible for the disappearance of the tumor, but do provide protection against subsequent infection. However, the antibodies were present in 65% of patients whose warts were cured, while they were present in only 23% of patients whose warts persisted.[28] It is thought that these IgG antibodies provide protection even in patients without prior infection, which may account for the declining incidence with increasing age.[149]

Ogilvie's studies suggested a relation between the appearance of circulating antiviral antibodies and the regression of the verrucae.[120] Genner reported that 6.3% of his subjects showed antibodies in complement-fixation reactions before therapy, whereas 20% showed them after therapy of some type.[60] Pass and associates demonstrated viral antigen in normal epidermis, but found it to be markedly increased in verrucae and a few other epidermal neoplasms; they believe this antigen is organospecific for epidermis.[124]

In 1972, Genner reported that the maximum antibody flouresence occurred in warts of 7 to 12 months duration, but was much less in warts of 18 months duration.[60] Pyrohonen and Pentlinen, who demonstrated antibody titers in 57% of their subjects with verrucae, also found that in older warts and in multiple warts, the antibody titer was lower. They theorized that this meant that: a) more antibodies are in use and thus the serum titer falls, or b) when antibody titers fall, the number and duration of warts increases.[135] These investigators also feel that the presence of IgG antibodies in a complement-fixation reaction indicates a healing period. It is therefore possible that the production of IgG antibodies by vaccination could be of value. In an effort to purify a wart-specific tissue antigen which related to the spontaneous involution of skin warts, Pass and Marcus recently discovered two antigens, a nuclear type and a cell-surface type.[125] They found these present in some other skin tumors and in minute quantities in normal skin.

It has been said that the future therapy for all "incurable" diseases lies in the understanding of immunology and its therapeutic applications. If medical science fails to discover a specific antiviral drug, verrucae may fall into this immunotherapy category. This approach is being studied experimentally.

Most investigators believe that the frequency of spontaneous resolution of warts reflects a successful immunologic response to the causative virus. Massing and Epstein reported that 2/3 of all types of verrucae in children involute spontaneously within two years.[104] Barr and Coles found a 20% incidence of spontaneous cures.[16] Children, in our experience, resolve in an average of six months. Horwitz and Marker discovered a 27% resolution of verrucae in patients on placebos in their study,[76] while Anderson and Shirreffs found over 60% cures with a placebo tablet.[9] Almeida and Goffe found that the recurrence of verrucae seemed to be associated with a lack of circulating antibody.[6] On this basis, they theorize that many of the current therapies destroy the virus before it can exert an antigenic stimulus (maximum antibody is found in warts of 7 to 12 months duration).[60] Is it possible that our rapid and thorough removal of verrucae may only leave the patient susceptible to recurrence and the growth of new wart colonies?

Clinical Considerations

The plantar wart and the common wart are similar. However, due to its location, the plantar wart is subject to pressure and tends to grow inward rather than protruding above the surface of the skin. Although verrucae are epidermal neoplasms, Matthewson has reported cases which, secondary to this pressure of weight-bearing, have enlarged inward through the dermis, subcutaneous tissue, and fascia.[105] Pressure and sheer forces also cause a considerable amount of hyperkeratotic (callus) tissue on the surface of the plantar wart, and usually a significant amount of pain. Pain is usually the chief complaint in verruca plantaris, while verruca vulgaris is usually just a cosmetic annoyance. Cancerphobia is not an uncommon reason for seeking consultation for warts. The onset and rate of growth of warts is usually more rapid than that of the other common hyperkeratotic skin lesions, especially in children.

A verruca is a true tumor and, therefore, shows none of the characteristics of normal skin such as skin lines, pinkness, which blanches on pressure, and uniform texture. There is usually a clear line of demarcation between the verrucous and normal tissue and the skin lines circumvent the tumor. The presence of more discomfort on lateral pressure (squeezing) than on direct pressure may differentiate a verruca from a flat callus, but not from a deep hyperkeratotic lesion, such as Steinberg's porokeratosis plantaris discreta.

The best gross diagnostic feature of verrucae are the minute bleeding points which are evident after paring away the hyperkeratotic surface of the wart. These bleeding points are the many fragile capillaries in the hyperplastic papillae, which extend abnormally high in the epidermis of all papillomas. This feature may be absent in older warts.[93]

Histopathology

Miscroscopically, verruca plantaris is a localized hyperplasia of epilthelial cells characterized by extensive hyperkeratosis alternating with porokeratosis and acanthosis,[103] and a thickened granular layer.[137] The diagnostic feature of papillomas is elongation and upward proliferation of the papillae into the epidermis. The lateral papillae tend to bend toward the center at the base of the lesion.[137] The basal epidermal layer is generally intact. Verrucae are differentiated from other papillomas by the presence of large, vacuolated cells in the upper stratum malpighian and in the granular layer; these may be absent in older warts.[93] The virus lives and replicates in the nucleus of these vacuolated cells, but is not evident in the basal layer, as in molluscum contagiosum. There may be a variable amount of inflammatory infiltrate present in the underlying upper or mid dermis.

Differential Diagnosis

As with any cutaneous neoplasm, differential diagnosis can only be confirmed histologically. However, an attempt will be made to offer gross clinical differences between verrucae and other similar lesions. Gibbs presented a good differential diagnosis of verruca plantaris in 1969.[62] The differentiation of common corns and calluses can only be made after the superficial layer of hyperkeratotic tissue is removed. A simple excrescence has a base of smooth waxy, non-granular, avascular stratum corneum with normal skin lines traversing across it. Porokeratosis of Steinberg shows the same subjective findings as verruca plantaris, and is similar in location and gross appearance; however, the central portion of porokeratosis plantaris discreta is smooth, non-granular, and does not present papillary bleeding points.[158]

Most skin tumors of the weight-bearing surface of the foot will have an armour of hyperkeratotic tissue similar to that of a plantar wart. Granulomas secondary to foreign body implantation, especially pet hairs, are not uncommon on the sole and often a good history will suggest this diagnosis. Epidermoid cysts appear grossly as a soft tissue mass underneath normal skin with or without a calloused surface. Eccrine poromas which are seen plantarly and occasionally interdigitally, are usually pedunculated and pink-to-red in color. Granuloma pyogenicum, an uncommon lesion of the foot, is generally raised and very vascular.

Amelanotic melanoma, although often asymptomatic, may appear grossly like a wart. Other malignant neoplasms are quite uncommon on the foot, but basal or prickle cell epithelioma and a single nodule of Kaposi's sarcoma must be ruled out. Shields and associates include in their differential diagnosis molluscum contagiosum.[149] Molluscum contagiosum on the plantar surface may take on a hyperkeratotic surface and be confused with that of the plantar wart; we have even confused a verrucous keratoacanthoma on the sole with a wart.

Henenfeld's treatise on the differential diagnosis of verruca plantaris included some of the less common lesions which resemble warts: pre-cancerous dermatoses, epidermodysplasia verruciformis, (called epithelial nevi or icthyosis hystrix), congenital hyperkeratosis and acanthosis (birthmarks), nevus verrucosa (focal keratosis), basosquamous cell acanthoma, fibroepithelial papillomas (non-viral), nodular hidradenomas, and cutaneous hematomas of the tuberous sclerosis syndrome.[73]

For many years pressure callosities were often misdiagnosed as plantar warts and treated by means not directed to the bony structural problem. This trend fortunately is reversing and radical surgical procedures such as the Dickson and Dively pie operation is frowned upon.

The following entities are mentioned in some detail because of their frequency on the foot. They are often misdiagnosed as plantar warts.

1. *Hyperkeratotic squamous papilloma* — This is an entity which closely resembles that of the plantar wart. The etiological factors are generally unknown, however, it may be due to a viral agent.

These lesions may vary in size from several millimeters to a centimeter in diameter. They may occur on any area of the plantar surfaces of the foot, and rarely do they occur on the dorsal surfaces of the foot. Grossly they may appear as small, round, or oval-shaped lesions similar to that of the verrucae. However, they have a much lighter appearance than the verrucae, and usually do not show any of the dark punctate areas from the capillaries as seen in plantar warts. In our personal experience they seem to occur more commonly in the thirty to sixty-year old age group, and are much less common than warts in the younger age group.

Signs and symptoms of hyperkeratotic squamous papilloma are identical to those of the plantar wart. In our clinical experience we have seen them spread on the sole.

Hyperkeratotic squamous papilloma has all the microscopic characteristics of the verrucae, except that viral inclusion bodies cannot be demonstrated. It is a possibility that these lesions may be burnt out warts in which viral replication is no longer taking place, or viral papillomas in which the replication virons simply do not assume the same staining characteristics as those of a true verrucae. It is also possible that these lesions may have possibly been plantar warts at an early stage, but, possibly due to constant weight bearing pressures, its true viral structures may have been lost. Certainly more investigation in this area is needed.

The treatment is identical to that of the plantar wart, with blunt surgical currettement establishing a very good surgical cure. Our experience, however, has revealed that the recurrence rate is much higher in hyperkeratotic papilloma than in the common plantar wart; cautery after excision has reduced its recurrence rate.

2. *Black Heel* — This is a condition which may closely resemble plantar warts. However, it is usually located on the lateral or

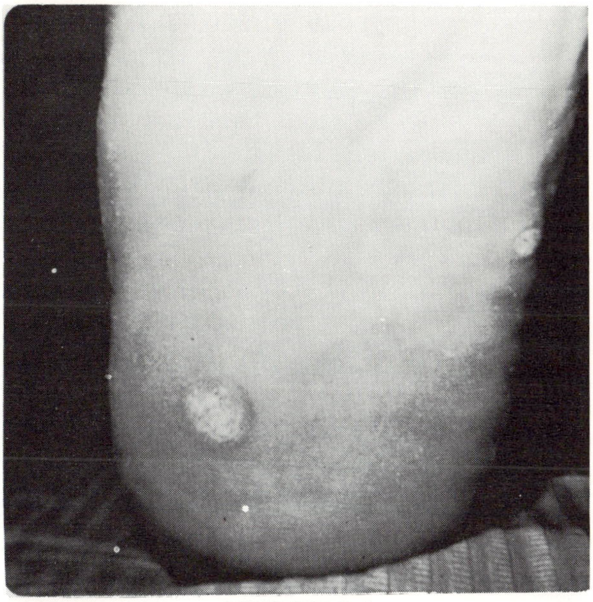

FIGURE 2-4

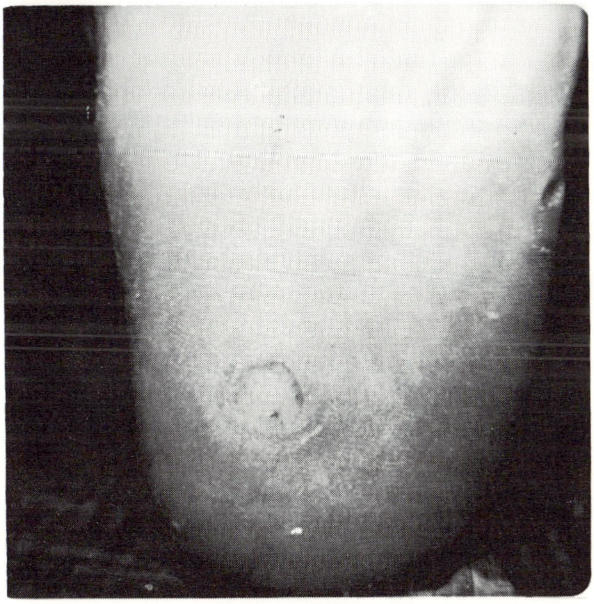

FIGURE 2-5

Hyperkeratotic Squamous Papilloma: Duration of lesion usually shows increase of hyperkeratosis and pigmentation. Photo's demonstrate before and after local debridement of hyperkeratotic tissue.

medial aspect of the heel, seen more frequently in the female, and is characteristic of local trauma tissue. We have also seen this condition on the medial plantar surface of the great toe. The darkened areas are probably from deposition of hemoglobin due to capillary or subepidermal bleeding. Treatment usually involves the removal of any additional trauma. These lesions are usually incidental findings and seldom present any symptoms or problems.

Treatment of Verruca

Medical literature is replete with reports on the merits of hundreds of remedies for verrucae, particularly verruca plantaris. Certainly, if any one therapy was a panacea, there would be no need to search so often for new methods. Although most authors report on acceptable percentage of cures for so stubborn a disease, few clinicians achieve the same success with the same treatment. In their discussion of warts, Prazak and Thomas summed it up: "The methods of the therapy reported in the literature seem to give good results in the respective author's hands, but the attempts of others to reproduce them often fail."[132]

Thus, a good method of treatment is one that is easily reproducible and has the best rate of success without recurrence in the literature. Of course, as with any therapy, the method must be adjusted to the state of the disease in the specific patient. On the topic of wart therapy, Samuel M. Peck said, "The best method is one you know best and the one which gives you the best results."[126] In an attempt to organize the myriad of reported treatments for verrucae, they have been classified under the following headings:

1. Psychotherapy
2. Roentgenotherapy
3. Cryotherapy
4. Topical Chemotherapy
5. Treatment using Electrical Modalities
6. Injectable Chemotherapy
7. Systemic Therapy
8. Surgical Therapy
9. Miscellaneous Treatments.

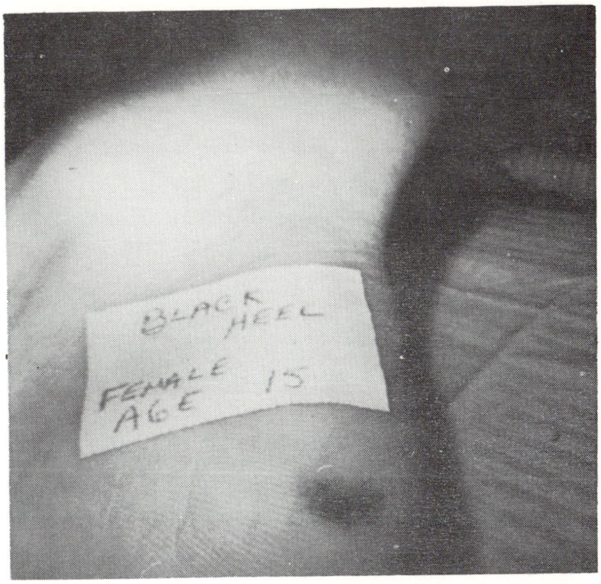

FIGURE 2-6

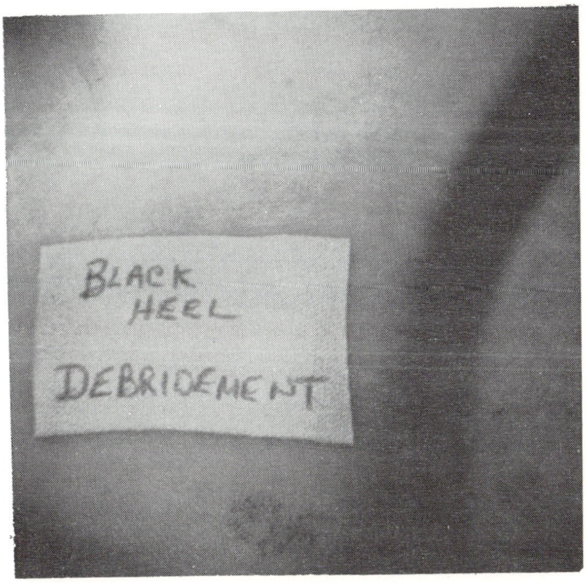

FIGURE 2-7

Black Heel: Often mis-diagnosed as a large verruca. Can be seen over most any pressure area of the foot. The heel is the most common area with the medial surface of the hallux toe and first metatarsal phalangeal joint seen on occasion.

1. Psychotherapy — A Review of the Literature

Allington presented the first good review of the psychotherapy of verruce in 1953.[4] According to Rulison, the average duration of all types of warts presented for therapy is about two years, three months, and 50% of 921 cases had a second attack.[143] He also stated that the area of inflammation around a wart just prior to spontaneous resolution suggests an antibody-antigen reaction.

Psychotherapy is usually carried out in combination with some form of placebo, such as saline injections, various functionless electrical machines, colorful paints and dyes, or an unplugged X-ray machine. Allington believes that the evidence of the efficacy of psychotherapy for warts is inconclusive.

Clarke stated in regard to psychotherapy, "The dramatic cures sometimes reported are probably the result of the magic ritual coinciding with the end of the warts' 'natural life'."[38] Clarke, like Allington, stresses the importance of the duration of the verruca because spontaneous cures occur in 40% to 88% of warts well over one year old, regardless of therapy.

Recently, Surman and associates tested the hypothesis that verrucae can be cured by hypnosis.[156] They found that warts do tend to respond to suggestion, with 53% improvement and 29% remission. Although this study supports Stankler, and Tenzel and Taylor in offering evidence that suggestion is a valid treatment for verrucae, these investigators stress that warts are not influenced selectively.[152,159] Montgomery supports the use of suggestion in young patients with verruca plantaris.[116] Allen believes statistics on psychotherapy are impressive until medical science gains a better understanding of the immunology of verrucae, the debate as to whether suggestion actually plays a part in the spontaneous resolution of warts cannot be settled.[1]

2. Roentgenotherapy

Montgomery reported the use of X-rays to treat verruca plantaris in 1929,[114] as did Goldsmith in 1936.[65] Since that time, many investigators have discussed the pros and cons of roentgenotherapy. In adequate doses, X-rays inhibit the hyperplastic cellular growth in epidermal neoplasms, and may also inhibit viral replication, although this has not been proven. The stagnant verrucous cells then undergo gradual autolysis.

The advantages of X-ray therapy are:

a. Usually only one treatment, and rarely more than five are required.
b. No pain or disability for the patient.
c. High percentages of cures in experienced hands.

The technique involves the use of a lead shield with an appropriately sized aperture to protect healthy tissue, and the use of variable roentgen-time-distance combinations.

The disadvantage of X-ray therapy is skin damage such as radiodermatitis, scarring and ulceration. This complication is so common that Montgomery lists radiodermatitis scars under "common lesions of the feet;"[117] numerous articles have been written regarding the surgical repair of these problems. The most frequent causes are excessive doses and X-ray treatment of previously radiated warts, which is contraindicated. Since the complications of this therapy can be worse than the original problem many authors have voiced their disapproval of X-ray therapy.[33,40,102,103,155] Certainly roentgenotherapy should be reserved for radiologists and dermatologists trained in its use.

3. Cryotherapy

The use of extreme cold to cause necrosis of epidermal growths was first introduced in 1899 by White, who used liquid air. Since then, two substances have become mainstays in the therapy of warts: solid carbon dioxide (snow) and liquid nitrogen.

The advantages of cryotherapy are:
a. No need for injections or anesthesia
b. Minimal disability
c. Minimal chance of scarring
d. Often only one treatment, seldom more than three, are required

The disadvantages are:
a. Burning sensation during application and thawing, usually about 15 minutes duration.
b. Often painful for a few hours to a few days, particularly with excessive weight bearing.
c. May not penetrate deep enough to freeze many older verrucae on the plantar surface.

Carbon Dioxide Snow — first introduced to the dermatotherapeutic armamentarium in 1907 by William Allen Pusey. CO_2 Snow reaches negative 89° Fahrenheit. The first step

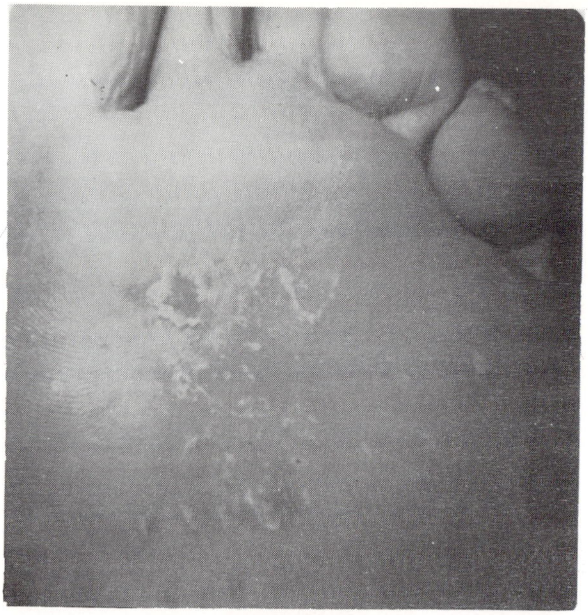

FIGURE 2-8

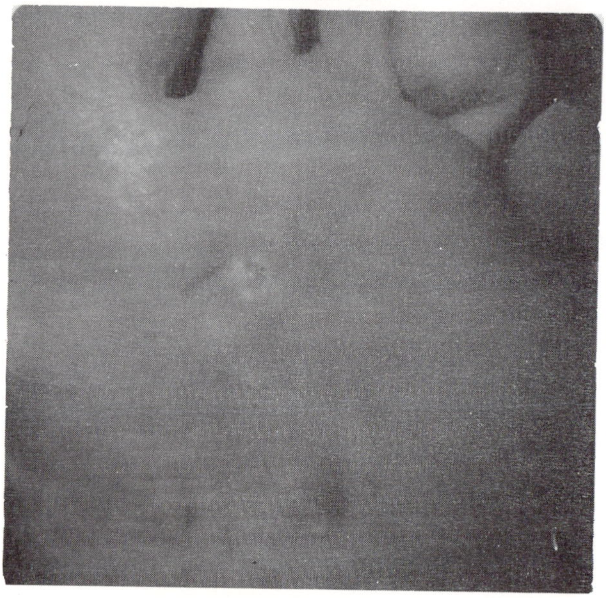

FIGURE 2-9

Radiation Scar: Radiation therapy can create much scarring and permanent disability. Often lesions under the metatarsal heads are mistaken for resistant verruca.

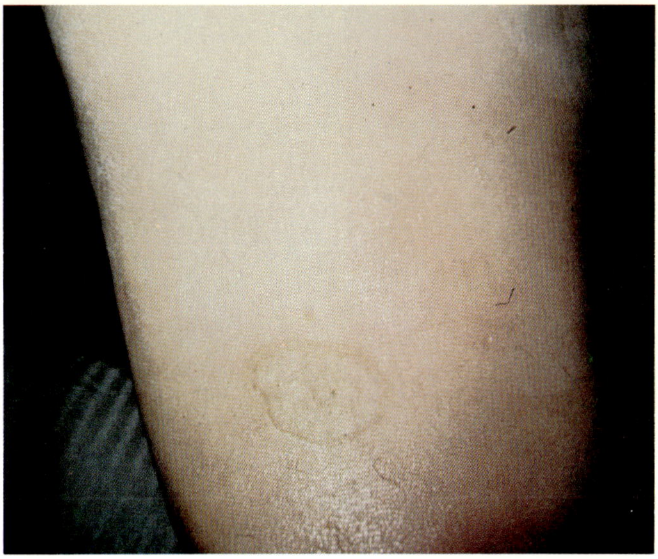

Mosaic Verruca — These lesions are the most difficult forms of plantar warts to treat, often affecting weight bearing surfaces. Pain on weight bearing is usually the most common symptom.

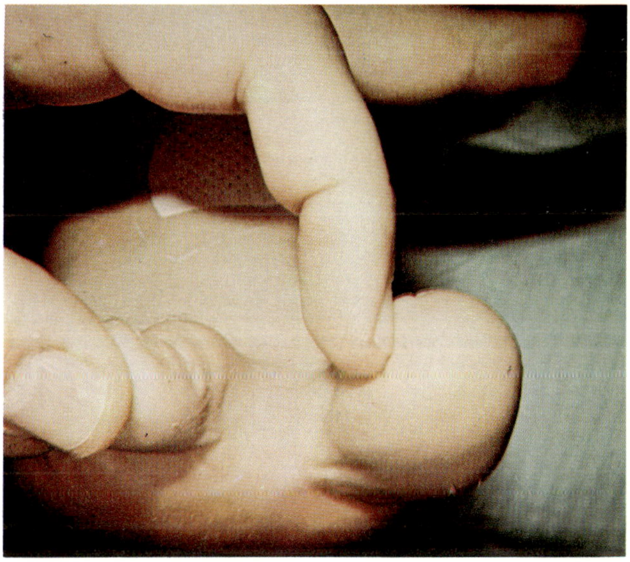

Interdigital Verruca — Warts are not common interdigitally. The diagnosis in this area is often difficult due to its lack of pigment and hyperkeratosis.

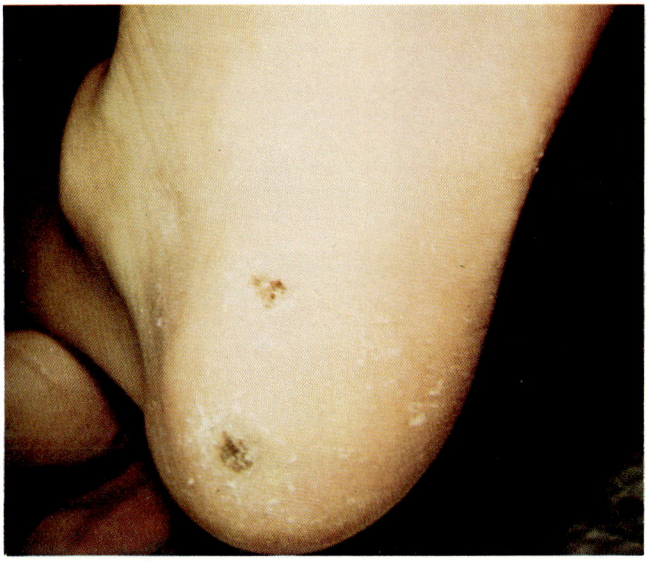

"Burnt-out" Wart — Plantar wart undergoing a self destruction process. These lesions become hemorhagic in color often presenting symptoms of discomfort. Etiology is unknown. Trauma and auto-immune processes may play a specific role.

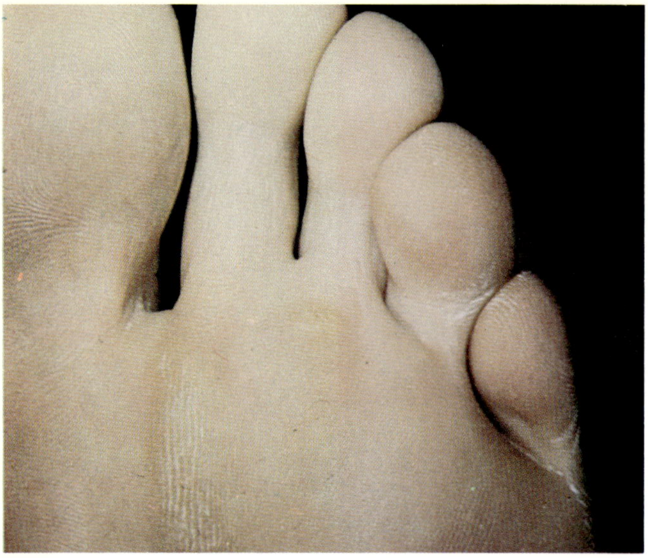

Hyperkeratotic Squamous Papilloma (Base of 3rd Toe) — These lesions are frequently seen on the sole and closely resemble the plantar wart both clinically and histologically.

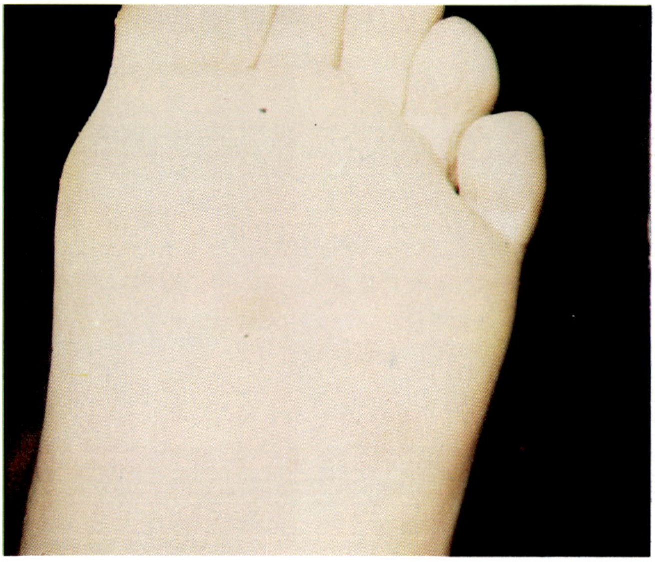

Molluscum Contagiosum — These lesions are early in development and are often confused with plantar warts. They occur with some frequency on the sole.

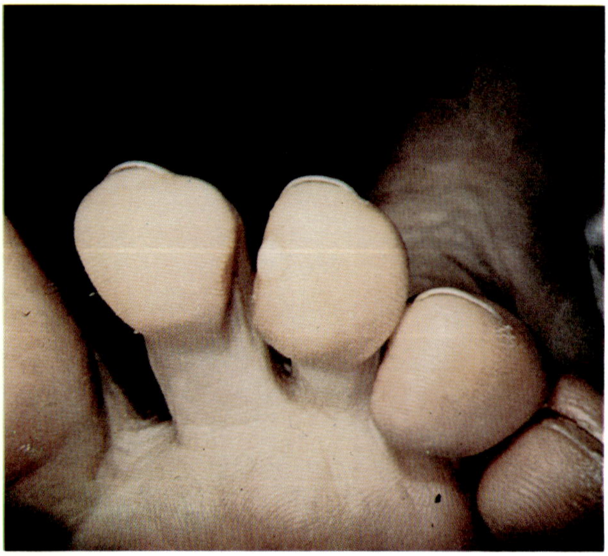

Hyperkeratosis with Fibrinoid Proliferation — Unusual hyperkeratotic lesion on distal aspect of digit. Clinically it appears as a fibrous tumor but histologically it is hyperkeratotic lesion.

in the method of application, according to Crow and Scott, is to pare down the hyperkeratotic armour until papillary bleeding is encountered.[43] Then the snow is applied with pressure, by means of special hollow "pencils" into which the CO_2 cylinder is injected, for a period of five minutes. This freezing results in a dermal-epidermal separation with subsequent bulla formation in about four days; if this blister is quite tender, it should be drained and dressed. Healing is complete in approximately one week. Crow and Scott reported a 93% cure with 7% recurrence in a series of 200 patients.[43]

Ignatoff recommends 60 second applications every two weeks for three treatments, and reports a 91% cure rate.[79] Montgomery, Shields and associates suggest CO_2 as a primary therapy, especially for children,[116,149] and Desforges recommends it in mosaic verrucae.[45] Kingland reported a 95% cure with one to four CO_2 treatments in 86 patients with plantar warts.[84]

Liquid Nitrogen — As described in 1950 by Allington, liquid nitrogen is stored in pyrex flasks at negative 319° F., and must be replaced weekly.[3] After the hyperkeratotic callus has been removed by paring or with salicylic acid plasters, Matthewson recommends applying the liquid nitrogen with a cotton swab for a period of about 15 minutes, and using pressure for deeper lesions.[105] In one week the resultant bulla is drained and the central stalk excised, and in another week the area is usually healed. Matthewson reports a cure in 62 of 63 patients. Goodman advocates liquid nitrogen, especially for periungual warts, but recommends a one to two minute application for one to three treatments.[66] Dorsey presents a bibliography of several authors who agree that cryotherapy has no advantage over other methods in plantar warts, whereas it is the method of choice in common warts.[49]

4. Topical Chemotherapy

Destruction of verrucous tissue by means of various keratolytic agents, such as acids and resins, is one of the oldest and continues to be one of the most popular treatments for verruca plantaris. Only chemicals which have been reported in the literature will be discussed here.

The advantages of topical therapy in general are:

a. No injection or anesthesia necessary.

b. Minimal disability
c. Minimal discomfort
d. Little chance of scarring.

The disadvantages are:

a. Usually requires several treatments.
b. Cure rate is quite variable due to difficulty in controlling the destruction.

Acids

Acids comprise the most frequently used treatments for plantar verrucae by the general medical public. Salicylic acid is usually used as a keratolytic as 40% or 60% in a cream or vaseline base. It is applied in the aperture of a pressure dressing. The verruca must be debrided and the dressing reapplied from one to several times to effect total destruction. Montgomery suggests this treatment weekly for mosaic verrucae.[117] Ecker recommends salicylic acid 60%, for three to four weeks before the surgeon resorts to plastic surgical repair.[52] Bunney reported the home use of a salicylic acid-lactic acid paint.[33] Ignatoff reported a 60% cure with the application of a salicylic acid and podophyllum resin suspension.[79] Lapidus recommends the use of 50% salicylic acid ointment covered with a 40% salicylic acid plaster on a weekly basis.[88]

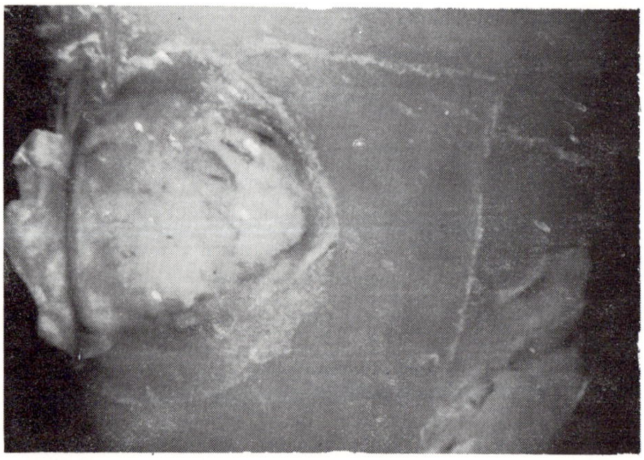

FIGURE 2-10

Mosaic Verruca: Large heel lesions and very resistant to therapy. Presently undergoing 60% Salicylic Acid Ointment treatment.

The active acids are frequently used in the drop form; Ignatoff reports a 75% cure ratio in five to eight weeks of therapy.[79] Perlstein utilized weekly applications of monochloracetic acid.[127] Woolf suggests the use of an exact amount (3/4″ in a 75 mm capillary tube) of trichloracetic acid, combined with multiple epidermal punctures, for two to three treatments.[172] The acids are often used in combinations. The "Blank Method" involves the use of one drop of 88% phenol (liquified carbolic acid) and one drop of fuming nitric acid, then a covering with 60% salicylic acid in petrolatum; Blank reported a 95% cure rate in four treatments.[19] Brady combines the use of Xine (Georges — 80% monochloracetic acid) applied with the multi-puncture technique, and a 60% salicylic acid dressing.[26] For periungual warts, Prozak and Lazar use full strength trichloroacetic acid followed by a 40% salicylic acid plaster and an occulsive dressing.[131] Carter suggests combining monochloroacetic acid and 50% silver nitrate with the use of oral Vitamin A.[34] Ignatoff also reports an 80% to 90% cure rate in four treatments with pyrogollic acid paste.[79] Recently, retinoic acid has proven beneficial in the treatment of flat warts, but its merit in treating verruca plantaris has not been established.

Other commonly used topical chemicals

Cantharidin is a strong vessicant (blister former) which is applied in a film forming vehicle. After the overlying callus is removed, a drop of cantharidin is applied, a film allowed to form, and then the wart is covered with non-porous tape. On the next visit, the bleb is drained and debrided, and any remaining verrucous tissue is touched with cantharidin. The specific advantage of this therapy is the limited number of treatments required; however, more pain than with other topicals is often encountered. Epstein and Kligman recommend Cantharone (Ingram) for periungual warts, but were not impressed with their achievement with plantar warts.[56]

Formalin U.S.P., which is 37% formaldehyde, is classified pharmacologically as a disinfectant and drying agent. Thomson introduced formalin as a therapy for verruca plantaris in 1943.[162] Formalin has been used most often (a) in combination with Aquaphor ointment, or (b) in a 3% to 27% solution as a soak. Therapy usually requires six to eight weeks. Glutaraldhyde can be substituted for formaldehyde, but it is less stable and more expensive.

Podophyllum resin, which has long been used as a treatment for condylloma acuminata (moist warts), was introduced as a therapy for verruca plantaris by Kurtin and Yontef in 1948.[86] Walz (1953) reported curing 11 of 13 plantar verrucae in one to ten treatments using 25% podophyllum in benzoin.[169] Manilla and associates recorded a 75% cure within 6 to 8 months using podophyllin ointment.[100] Thomson and Ormand stated that podophyllin often causes excessive pain, and thus do not recommend its use. [121,162]

Less Commonly used Topical Chemicals

Carslow and Neill presented an interesting therapy utilizing linseed oil in 1963.[33] They suggest that the main obstacle to the clearance of a plantar wart is its amount of keratin, which derives its hardness from the number of disulfide bonds (s-s) in its polypeptide chain. If you introduce an s-h group inhibitor, such as 70% unsaturated linseed oil, it should reduce the keratogenous zone to a soft, structureless substance. They achieved the best results (84.6% cure) with one application of the following (left dry for 7 days and intact for up to 12 weeks): Linseed oil, 20%; podophyllin resin, 20%, and lanolin, q.s. No further references to this therapy in the literature could be found.

Several British authors described the use of "nobecutane D" combined with formaldehyde with good results.[149,163] Manilla and associates discussed the daily use of Odpocirodome (Allergan Pharmaceuticals) 0.5% in Aquaphor base for one month, and reported excellent results.[101] Brezak tried topical clethacimjin with only fair results.[25] Ignatoff includes euphorbium resin in alcohol in his discussion of verruca therapy.[79]

Newer Topical Agents

Involution of warts following an acute allergic contact dermatitis in the area can be artificially induced by applying a potent allergen such as DNCB (2,4 - dinitrochlorobenzene). Bleamycin and 5 - fluourourocil are two anti-tumor, anti-DNA drugs which, when applied topically to warts, have shown promising clinical results.

5. Treatment Utilizing Electrical Modalities

Of the five forms of electrosurgery, electrodessication or fulguration is the least destructive and the safest for use on epidermal neoplasms.[146] An Oudin current producing a spark from a single electrode produces a charring of tissues; examples are the Hyfrecator and Bovie machines. The advantage of electro-surgery is that generally only one treatment is involved. The disadvantages are:

a. An injection of local anesthesia is necessary.
b. Moderate post-operative pain may be present.
c. The depth of the charring is difficult to control, too little voltage causing viable wart tissue to remain, while too much voltage can lead to destruction of deeper layers and subsequent scarring.

Katz suggested the use of electrodessication in 1948.[83] Monroe reported in 1956 that full-thickness fulguration of verrucae for one or two treatments was effective in 65% of patients over 20 years of age, and in 85% of patients under 20.[113] Silverman supported the use of fulguration in mosaic verrucae because he believes that the increase in temperature and acidity inhibits viral growth and replication by enzyme inhibition.[150]

In 1968, Smiler presented a good discussion of electrolysis, or negative galvanism, in the treatment of verruca plantaris.[151] The technique requires no anesthesia, and involves two insertions of a sterile, needle-like electrode through the base of the wart and parallel to the skin. He reported success in 50 cases. Ignatoff professes a 90% cure with electrodessication, but warns of the possibility of scar formation; he does not support the use of electrolysis.[79] Horwitz and Marken report a 55-60% cure rate with electrocautery.[76]

In 1962, Grady presented an interesting treatment for plantar warts.[68] Under local anesthesia, the verrucous tissue is "ground out" using a large steel burr and a high speed moto-drill. A compression dressing is required to control the profuse bleeding with this technique.

Ultrasound

The concept of eliminating warts by the use of ultrasonic therapy was introduced by Kent in 1959. Ultrasound therapy has the advantage of being quite non-traumatic; however, it usually involves many and frequent treatments.

Rowe and Gray state, "Whether the therapeutic effect of ultrasound in treating warts is due to heat, psychotherapy, or some other mechanism is not apparent at this time."[140] They utilize weekly treatments of 0.6 watts per cm^2 for 15 minutes. In their first series, they obtained a cure in 22 of 25 patients in 6 to 15

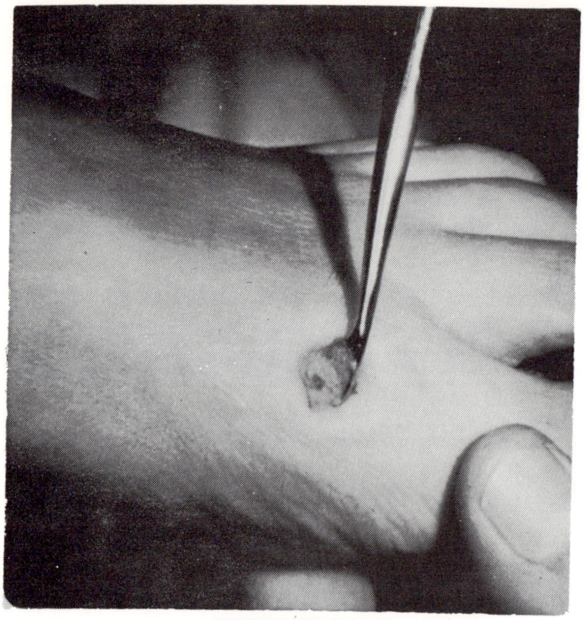

FIGURE 2-11

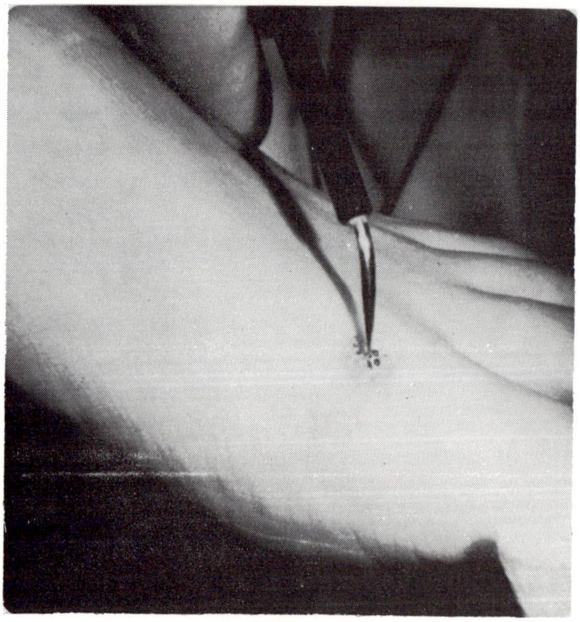

FIGURE 2-12

Verruca: Demonstration of dorsal wart undergoing blunt dissection and electrodessication.

treatments;[140]in their second series, they cured 84 of 100 patients, with half requiring less than 10 treatments and half needing 10 to 15 treatments.[141]

Manilla and associates found that ultrasound cured about 50% of verrucae after 20 to 30 treatments.[100] Recently, Vaughn compared direct and underwater treatment of plantar warts.[35 162] With the direct method, he obtained 83% disappearance and 97% relief of symptoms in an average 7 to 8 treatments; with the underwater method, he found 51% of warts disappeared and 88% had relief of symptoms, in an average 6 to 16 treatments.

There is some evidence that heat causes either a thermal activation of the wart virus and activates the immune process, or the heat slows the growth of the virus. LaCricchie and Haservick found that a 45-48° C. water bath comprised the most heat that their subjects could withstand that penetrated to the basal layer of the skin.[96] After three months of weekly 30 to 90 minute treatments, 9 to 15 patients had regression or disappearance of their warts; most patients complained of discomfort during treatments. The authors also question whether the water provides the cure rather than the heat — Anderson and Shirreffs found a 60% cure rate with plain water soaks.[9]

6. Injectable Chemotherapy

The intralesional or sublesional injection of different chemical agents to cure verrucae was initiated by Shellow, in 1934, using local injections of bismuth.[148] This study was followed by those of Demeur and Buske.[30,44] Buske reported in 1963, that he combined sublesional injection of bismuth cevitamate with local applications of Solisacan and oral bistrimate (bismuth triglycollamate — Smith, Miller and Patch, Inc.).[31] In 1953, Cohen expressed his opinion that bismuth therapy is useless.[39]

Ormond, also reported the local injection of bismuth sodium tartrate combined with local applications of 4% formaldehyde in aquaphor,[121] but later substituted an injectable sclerosing agent, 3% Sotredecol (Wallace and Tierman).[122]

The intra-epidermal injection of a local anesthetic under pressure to cause pressure necrosis and vascular insult to the verruca, was introduced in 1953 by Branson and Rhea, who utilized 2 to 3 cc's of 1% procaine.[23] Carpenter reported curing 67.5% of 217 plantar verrucae with one sublesional injection of about 1.8 cc of

2% anesthetic with epinephrine 1:100,000.[32] An added advantage to this therapy, according to Carpenter, is that the patient leaves the office completely asymptomatic. Stern discussed the use of Quinocaine (Farmsworth Pharm.), a long-acting anesthetic (3-21 days) which causes superficial necrosis in the epidermis.[154] In single verrucae, he found 95% were cured 3 to 5 weeks after one injection, while 30% of those patients with multiple verrucae required a second injection. The one disadvantage with this therapy is the possibility of hematoma formation and considerable pain after approximately three days.

Cramer reported the intralesional injection of an intramuscular trypain, Parenzymme (National Drug), with the main result being excessive pain.[42] Hyman noted that the sublesional injection of papain also caused a painful bulla to form.[78]

In 1956, Steinberg published the results of his study utilizing sublesional injections of a vitamin A solution, Keramin (Campbell Pharm. Co.).[153] Utilizing local anesthesia in two to eight injections, he found only 7 failures and no recurrences in 300 treatments. Gilbert and Williams used Steinberg's technique and achieved 82% cure and 95% improvement on 100 patients.[63] Lehman and Manning obtained 70% cures in 208 patients with three to five injections of Vitamin A,[91] and Klauder cured 30 of 31 patients with two to thirteen injections of Keramin.[85]

Ignatoff also lists some other sclerosing agents used in verruca therapy: 5% etharol in 2% procaine, 1-6% benzyl alcohol in 2% procaine, Varisol (Abbott),[79] and sodium moruate 5% in 2% procaine. He was impressed with the success of injection therapy, but stressed that injections, particularly in the plantar skin, are painful and usually must be repeated a few times to effect a cure.

7. Systemic Therapy

Systemic therapy for verrucae is either aimed at killing the virus in vivo or exciting an antigen-antibody reaction to destroy the virus.

A few studies regarding the use of the antimalarial, chloroquin, gave variable results: Murphy found that the cure rate was about the same (39%) in patients taking hydroxychloroquine sulfate and those taking a placebo.[118]

Biberstein and other workers were the first to attempt immunization therapy for verrucae. Biberstein injected a crude wart autolysate intracutaneously as a vaccine, twice weekly for 7 to 10 weeks, with nearly 75% cures.[18]

In another attempt to cure warts by simulating other antiviral therapies, Sakuranne and Sugan (1960) administered 0.1 grams of gamma globulin intradermally in the forearm twice weekly for an average of six weeks; they claim to have cured 28 of 32 verrucae.[144] However, it is doubtful that this therapy would lead to a significantly high enough plasma level of gamma globulin to have any effect on an intraepidermal neoplasm such as a verruca.

In the late 1960's, several authors (Allyn, McGee, Hutchinson, and Thompson) reported treating verruca plantaris by intralesional innoculation of unattenuated smallpox (vaccinia) vaccine by the multipuncture technique.[5,77,109,116] In these studies, the cure rate was uniformly good; however, morbidity in the form of pain, lymphangitis and fever was marked in 20% to 60% of the subjects.

The Committee on Cutaneous Health and Cosmetics of the American Medical Association disapproves of the use of direct innoculations of smallpox vaccine for treatment of verrucae because the morbidity rate is high.[8] They state that, "It is doubtful that the vaccinia virus has any direct antagonistic effect on the wart virus."

In a good review of this therapy, Lawrence reported treating 112 patients with a routine smallpox vaccination in the arm, and curing 67%; no adverse reactions were noted.[90] Lawrence and Anglin stress that any therapy using smallpox vaccine is contraindicated in patients not previously vaccinated as infants (most pediatricians now are not vaccinating infants for smallpox).[12]

8. Surgical Therapy

Two types of surgical therapy are commonly employed for plantar verrucae: a) curettage, a primary therapy for any verrucae, and b) plastic surgery, as a secondary therapy for intractable verrucae or the complications of previous therapies, including scarring and ulceration.

Hertz first discussed using a spoon-shaped instrument to remove plantar warts in 1948.[74]

Prazak and Thomas presented curettage as a means of eliminating verruca plantaris in 1955.[132] The technique, performed under local anesthesia, involves circumscribing the wart shallowly with a knife, and then, using a combination of prying and scraping motions, "scooping-out" the verruca with a Spratt bone curette, down to the basal-fascial layer only. They suggest using magnification to find and eradicate all verrucous projections. A five year follow-up yielded good results in this study. Prazak and Thomas stress the fact that this therapy is easily reproducible and provides the most visible evidence that the wart has been eliminated.

Lerner discussed the curettage of plantar warts using a mastoid curette,[92] as suggested by Weinstock,[170] and dressing the remaining cavity with a Gelfoam sponge (Upjohn), as per Overcast.[123] Lerner reported 91% success with a 9% recurrence, and he stressed that this therapy gives a good percentage of cures in the hands of any physician. Bornstein, Schenkman, Lauie, and McLaoughlin also recommend curettage for this reason.[22,89,110,147]

Antahades suggested utilizing a CO_2 applicator to freeze and demarcate the verrucae, as well as providing hemostasis, and curetting the verrucae quickly before sensation returns.[13]

Vickers related that the disadvantage to curettage was a 30% recurrence rate.[167] Suppan and Besterman suggested that after curetting down to the basal layer (which is pink tissue with skin lines — avoid reaching the fat globules of subcutaneous tissue), the base of the cavity should be swabbed with 88% phenol for three to five minutes to destroy any remaining verrucous cells, and the area dressed utilizing an enzyme-steroid ointment. They report a 95.7% cure with no recurrences.[150]

To accomplish plastic repair of refractory or complicated plantar verrucae, earlier authors advocated a cross-leg pedicle graft from the calf of the opposite leg, or Dickson's excision of the entire metatarsal-phalangeal ray.[106] Subsequent authors (Robinson, Monroe, and Conuag) suggested trying a full thickness homograft, the digital filleting procedure of Greeley,[40,113,138] or the digital shortening procedure of Giannini.[61] The latter two procedures involved using the skin of an adjoining digit to cover the plantar defect.

McQuire recommended using a full-thickness pedicle flap graft to place plantar skin over the weight-bearing area, and then using a full-thickness graft from the groin to cover the donor

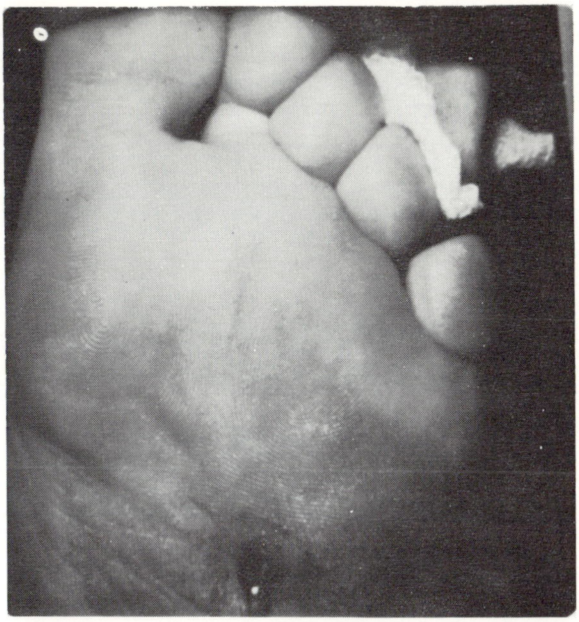

FIGURE 2-13

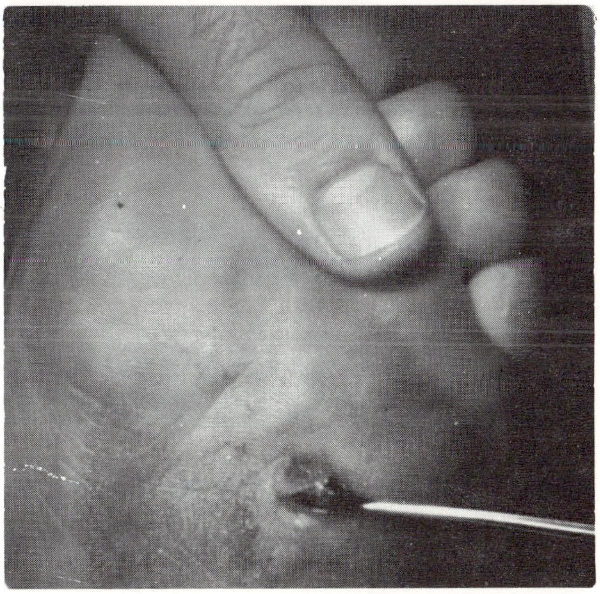

FIGURE 2-14

Plantar Wart: Photo demonstrates blunt dissection with bone currette. This is usually followed with chemical cautery.

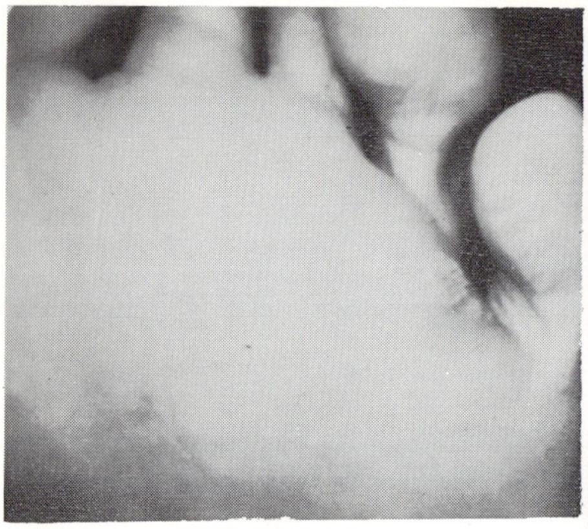

FIGURE 2-15

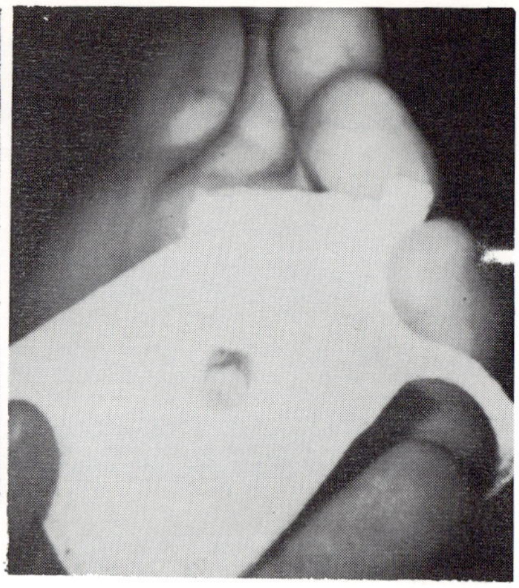

FIGURE 2-16

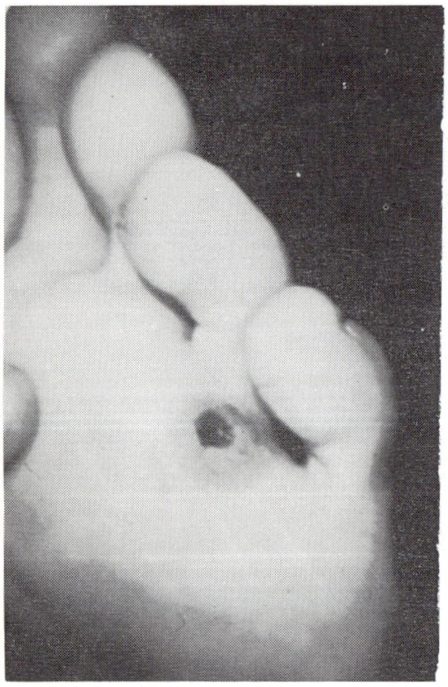

FIGURE 2-17

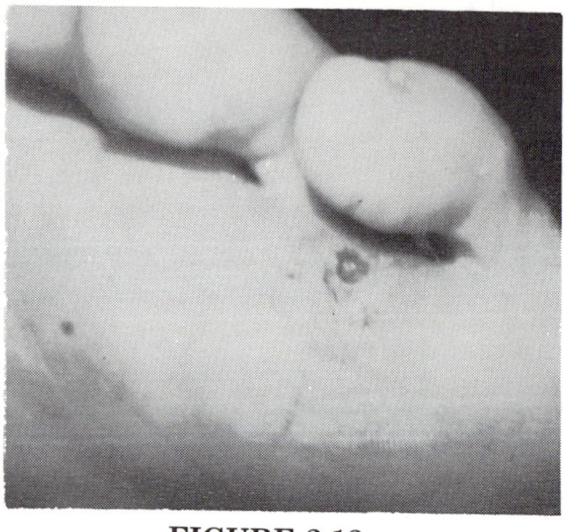

FIGURE 2-18

Plantar Wart: Blunt dissection of wart revealing lesion after excision. Figures 17 and 18 reveal the foot day of excision and week post-operative.

site.[111] Anderson combined this rotated pedicle graft with the plantar condylectomy of DuVries and cured 14 of 15 patients.[11,51] Dingman and Grabb suggested that the formula for successful plastic repair of these lesions is to: a) eliminate the ulcer, b) remove a portion of the underlying bone, and c) cover the defect with plantar skin.[46]

9. Miscellaneous Treatments

Utilizing orthopedic padding, strappings and orthotics to relieve the symptoms of plantar verrucae was advocated by Eden in 1952, who also believed that balance therapy occasionally cures these warts.[53] Rook recommends correcting any orthopedic defects in conjunction with other therapies for plantar warts to relieve symptoms and prevent recurrence.[139]

To treat shallow plantar verrucae in children, Boker reported success by using a five minute soap and brush scrubbing to the area nightly for three to six weeks.[14] For adults with verruca plantaris, Perreira-Marques suggests nightly soaking in 20% salt water followed by a salt water dressing covered with a plastic wrap to be worn throughout the night. When continued for four to eight weeks, this therapy yielded good results.[128]

Complications

The most frequent complications of verrucae are:

a. The establishment of new colonies ("Mother-Daughter") warts.
b. Recurrence following therapy.
c. Scarring or ulceration as a result of over-zealous treatment.

The multiplicity of reports regarding the plastic surgical repair of scars and ulcers resulting from attempts at irradiation of the plantar wart indicate the frequency of this complication. The most frequent cause of these scars is excessive doses of roentgen rays. Gardner and Acker reported the destruction of the distal phalanx of a thumb as a result of longstanding periungual warts. They believe this is the first reported case of verrucous tissue causing bony damage.[59]

Prognosis

The prognosis is often good but in many instances its success for any treatment can be frustrating to the patient and clinician.

Unfortunately most podiatrists and physicians never seem to cure certain individuals.

Statistics on the prognosis of verrucae without treatment are scarce. Conversely, statistics cited early in this chapter demonstrate the frequency of the spontaneous resolution of warts without therapy.[16,76,104]

In 1961, Anderson reported a 10-year follow-up study of 128 college students who were treated for verruca plantaris by various means (which were not mentioned). He found that 21 patients had recurrences or new growths within six months, and 52 had recurrences or new growths within 10 years; an estimated 20% of the warts were of the "therapy-resistant" type. In most cases, faster recurrence paralleled more resistance.

Molluscum Contagiosum

Molluscum contagiosum is a small, discrete, waxy, pearly white to grayish lesion with a central depression often darker in color. These benign tumors are often multiple and may range in number from one to twenty. It is a self-limiting viral disease and the tumors usually resolve without scarring in 6 to 9 months.[139] The name molluscum is from the latin for "soft", which implies that these are soft tumors of a contagious nature.

Etiology and General Considerations

Molluscum contagiosum is a mildly contagious viral disease of the skin. The incubation period is reported to be from 14 days to 12 months.[129] Studies by Goldschmidt and Kligman indicate that the virus may be widely distributed in the stratum spinosum of normal skin for many years without exciting a host response or clinical infection.[64] Juliusberg first suspected a viral etiology in 1905, when his innoculation of tumor extracts into normal skin caused lesions in two to seven weeks.

Pox virus mollusci is a brick-shaped, ectodermotropic virus. It is one of the largest viruses known to infect humans.[97] It has rarely been transmitted experimentally.[101] Prose, et al, have transferred the pox virus to tissue cultures of normal skin; they found that the virus particles were ingested within phagocytic vacuoles in the cytoplasm where they remained unchanged and unreplicated.[133] In infected cells, the replication is introcytoplasmic.[15]

Circulating antibodies to the molluscum virus were found by fluorescence microscopy in 87% of infected patients by Epstein, et al.[55] However, subjects continually exposed to infected patients do not develop antibodies. The antigenic substance involved was discovered by immunoflourescence in the cytoplasmic inclusion bodies.

Onset

Molluscum contagiosum may occur in any age, but the peak incidence is in children from 10 to 15 years old. Small epidemics have been reported in mental institutions for youths. Falknor reported three cases in children on the dorsum of the foot in which the trauma of walking barefoot was the common denomination.[57] Henas and Freeman reported an atypical case of inflammatory molluscum contagiosum as a result of the contents of the papule being discharged into the dermis.[72]

Review of the Literature

Most authors state that molluscum contagiosum is rare on the sole. Baxter and Carsen claim to have reported the first case.[17] Bunney believes that molluscum contagiosum of the sole usually remains undiagnosed due to its slightly uncharacteristic appearance as a result of weight bearing pressure; it is probably more common on the soles than formerly believed.[29]

Our personal experience has shown these lesions to be relatively common, often being confused with plantar warts. We have experienced many cases as a primary complication after surgical currettement of warts, where they would appear two to four weeks post-operatively. Thus, there may be a possibility that the wart and molluscum virus are related or, it may be, coincidentally present, or the pox virus may be lying dormant in the epidermis and be stimulated by the previous therapy.

Histological Appearance

Molluscum tumors are papules of acanthotic epidermis which occasionally show hyperkeratosis and parakeratosis.[175] They may impinge upon or extend into the dermis initiating hyperemia and lymphocytosis. Large, eosinophilic viral inclusion bodies are usually seen in vacuolated cytoplasm; the most frequent site is the cells of the stratum malpighii.[157] These inclusion bodies are so characteristic that they are referred to as "molluscum bodies."[17]

Differential Diagnosis

Lichen planus presents multiple, pruritic papules similar to molluscum contagiosum, except that the former lesions are usually violaceous in color. Verruca vulgaris and plantaris are also similar, but are papillomatous after paring with a sharp blade. Foreign body granuloma and eccrine poroma are rarely multiple, and keratoacanthoma and basal cell carcinoma are rare on the foot.

Treatment

Treatment of molluscum contagiosum is aimed at relieving symptoms and preventing contagion, because resolution of the tumors is spontaneous in a period of months. Currettage, under local anesthesia, may be the best form of treatment. Liquid nitrogen or phenol application is a less traumatic therapy for multiple lesions. Recurrence after therapy is not uncommon. Some broad spectrum antibiotics have a static effect on the growth of very large viruses, and thus have produced some good but variable results in cases of molluscum contagiosum. Oxytetracycline has affected some cures.

Herpes Simplex

Herpes simplex is a viral infection of the skin which is usually asymptomatic and may present itself as a vessicular eruption of the skin and mucous membranes. This viral infection is usually seen in the upper extremities, particularly around the lips, head, face and genitalia. It is usually the recurrent lesions that one may see on the extremities and particularly, the foot. The primary lesions may first demonstrate themselves in individuals under the age of five, and often there is some systemic reaction such as fever, and malaise, lasting about 10-14 days.

Etiology

The etiology is the herpes virus hominis. However, recurrence of these herpes simplex lesions may be brought about by fever, sunlight, trauma, food, drugs, and emotional stress. There are two distinct types of herpes simplex. Type I are lesions characteristically seen above the waist; Type II are lesions located below the waist.

Clinical Picture

The clinical appearance on the foot is generally the same as other glabrous skin areas, but it is very unusual to see them on the foot. It may present itself as a group of small, clear vessicles, which subsequently dry and form crusts. Healing generally takes place in about ten days, usually resulting in no scar formations. According to Samitz and Dana, there are two specific forms of herpes simplex which may occur on the foot:

1. Innoculation herpes simplex - herpes simplex believed to develop in an area with a history of injury.
2. Eczema Herpeticum — superimposed herpes simplex infection in a patient with a previous dermatitis.

In association with these lesions on the foot, one may also have pain and associated lymphangitis which may present itself as a pyogenic infection. Herpetic whitlows may also occur on the digits, however, these are extremely rare on the toes. They are often seen on the fingers in various occupations such as dentists, dental assistants and nurses, with housewives comprising the largest individual group.[54] There appears to be no differentiation between the sexes and herpes simplex may occur at any season, with the summer months most common.[54]

Differential Diagnosis

Pemphigus vulgaris.

Treatment

Prophylaxis: Since certain stimuli may predispose itself to a recurrent form of herpes simplex, prevention of sunburn due to ultra-violet radiation should be encouraged. Emotional tension should also be decreased. Any of the etiologic stimuli in the presentation of herpes simplex should be avoided if at all possible. In the treatment of the primary infection, supportive systemic therapy is very important. Simple measure, however, may be applied such as drying lotions in the early vesicular, or the oozing stages of the disease. After the drying of such blisters, various lubricating ointments may also be applied which may prevent cracking and also soften the crusted appearance of the lesion. Antibiotic therapy may also be necessary to prevent the possibility of a secondary bacterial infection. Recently, the use of special dyes and exposure to a fluorescent light have been used.

Herpes Zoster (Shingles)

Herpes Zoster is usually a localized viral disease exemplified by painful circumscribed vessicular eruptions which may also present itself with concurrent inflammation of the associated dorsal root, or extramedullary cranial nerve ganglions.

Etiology

The etiology is the herpes zoster virus which is identical to that of the varicella (chickenpox) virus.

Clinical Picture

These lesions may vary in size from several millimeters to reaching a centimeter in diameter. They may occur on any area of the plantar surfaces of the foot. Incubation period of the varicella — zoster virus is unknown. Papulovessicular lesions may occur on one or more dermatomes of the skin. Shortly afterwards, crops of vessicles and maculopapular plaques develop. These vessicles are usually clear, but become purulent with crust formation. This process may last from one to five weeks. The primary crusted lesions usually present themselves with no scarring from normal healing. However, if secondary infection does take place, scarring may result. This condition is most often unilateral.

Signs and Symptoms

Pain is the most common feature in this viral disease. However, itching, fever, and generalized G.I. symptoms may also present themselves. The infection involves one or more dermatomes of the skin, supplied by the dorsal nerve root or extramedullary cranial nerve ganglions, and is usually accompanied by pain. Herpes zoster is rarely seen on the foot, and generally reveals pustular type lesions. These lesions often undergo crusting. The lesions may last anywhere from two to four weeks, however, persistent post zosteriform pain may be troublesome for many months, and in rare instances even disabling for several years, particularly in older individuals.

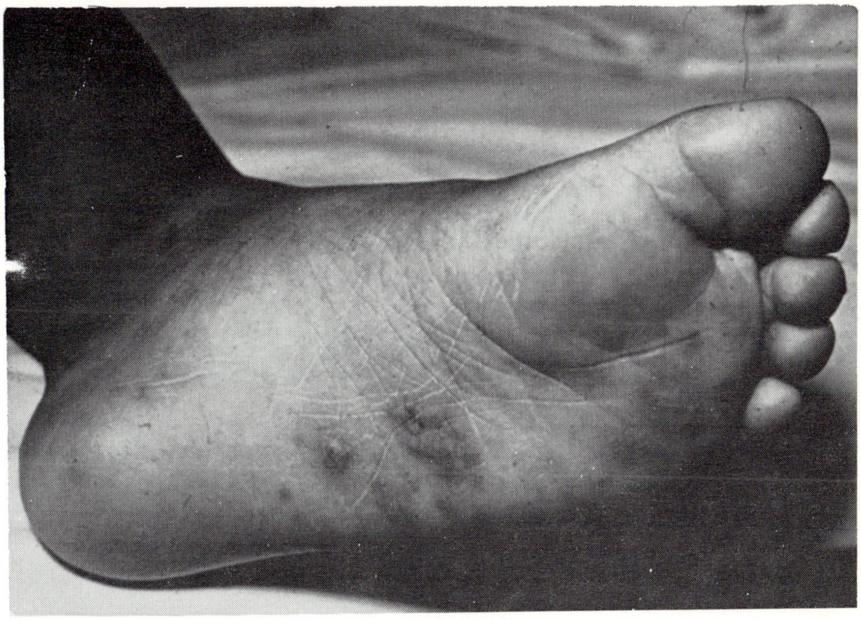

FIGURE 2-19

Herpes Zoster: Invariably unilateral, only rarely seen below the knee. Neuritic pain is prominent in at least 2/3 of patients, but in young children may be slight or absent. (Courtesy William V. R. Shellow, M.D., Los Angeles, Calif.)

Laboratory Diagnosis

Diagnosis of herpes simplex and herpes zoster can be made in differentiation by 1) isolation of the virus from the vessicle content, 2) the study of flourescent antibodies, and 3) other serologic methods.[58] Other diagnostic tests for viral infections of the foot can be demonstrated by evaluating the viral particles in vessicle fluid, usually under electron-microscope, and punch biopsy.[58]

Differential Diagnosis

Differential diagnosis includes hand, foot, and mouth disease; herpes simplex; contact dermatitis; and tinea pedis.

Complications

Complications involving lower extremity paralysis are quite rare in this condition. Broadbent, in 1866, presented the first case of a paralytic extremity due to zoster. This case, however, involved the upper extremity.[142] Lal has reported a specific case involving a foot drop with painful vessicles appearing a day or two after the patient's complaint was evaluated.[87]

Treatment

Treatment today is that of supportive care, usually in the relief of pain, and isolation of the individual in the vessicle stages to prevent a spread to others. The skin lesions, particularly those of the foot are treated with wet to dry compresses usually being cool in nature and having astringent properties. After the lesions have completely dried, the applications of steroid creams or even antibiotic ointments may also be utilized. Systemic corticosteriods are frequently used in the early course of the disease to relieve pain and to prevent zosteriform pain in older age groups.

BIBLIOGRAPHY

1. Allen, A. C.: *The Skin,* 2nd ed. Grune & Stratton, New York, 1967.
2. Allen, W. H. and Dickson, V. A.: An etiologic study of verruca plantaris. *Med. Offr.,* **119**:261, 1968.
3. Allington, H. V.: Liquid nitrogen therapy for warts. *Cal. Med.,* **72**:153, 1950.
4. Allington, H. V.: Review of psychotherapy of warts. *Arch. Derm. Syph.,* **66**:316-326, 1952.
5. Allyn, B., et al: Treatment of verruca with vaccina. *JAMA,***230**:807, 1968.
6. Almeida, J. A. and Goffe: Antibody to wart virus in human sera demonstrated by electron microscopy and precipitin texts. *Lancet,* **2**:1205-1207, 1965.
7. Almeida, J. D., Howatson, A. F., and Williams, M. G.: Electron microscope study of human warts. *J. Invest. Derm.,* **38**:337-345, 1962.
8. A.M.A. — C.C.H.C.: Treatment of warts with smallpox vaccine. *JAMA,* **206**:117, 1968.
9. Anderson, I. and Shirreffs, E.: The treatment of plantar warts. *Brit. J. Derm.,***75**:29-32, 1963.
10. Anderson, P. C.: Recurrence of verruca plantaris after destruction. *U. Mich. Med. Bull.,* **27**:286-288, 1961.
11. Anderson, R.: The treatment of intractable plantar warts. *Plast. Reconstr. Surg.,* **19**:384-388, 1957.
12. Anglin, C. S.: An adverse reaction from treating warts with vaccinia virus. *Canad. Med. Assoc. J.,* **99**:119-121, 1968.
13. Antahades, L. M.: Refrigeration anesthesia in the surgical excision of a plantar wart, a case report. *JAMA,* **53**:662-663, 1963.
14. Baker, H.: Another treatment for plantar warts in children. *Canad. Med. Assoc. J.,* **85**:1206, 1961.
15. Banfield, W. G. and Bridley, D. C.: An electron microscopic study of the epidermal lesions of molluscum contagiosum. *Ann. N.Y. Acad. Sci.,* **81**:145-163, 1959.

16. Barr, A. and Coles, R. B.: The natural history of warts. *Trans. St. Johns Hosp. Derm. Soc.,* **52**:226, 1966.
17. Baxter, D. L. and Carsen, J.: Molluscum contagiosum of the sole. *Arch. Derm.,* **89**:471-472, 1964.
18. Biberstein, H.: Immunization therapy of warts. *Arch. Derm. Syph.,* **46**:66, 1942.
19. Blank, H.: Treatment of plantar warts. *Arch. Derm. Syph.,* **56**:446-459, 1947.
20. Blank, H.: Virus-induced tumors of human skin. *N.Y. Acad. Sci.,* **54**:1226-1231, 1952.
21. Blank, H. and Rake, G.: Warts (chapter IX) *Viral and Rickettsial Diseases of Man,* Churchill, London, 1955, pp. 156-181.
22. Bornstein, B.: Effects of oral chymotrysin on surgical sequelae. *JAPA,* **53**:349-351, 1963.
23. Branson, E. C. and Rhea, R. L.: Plantar warts: Cure by injection. *New Eng. J. Med.,* **248**:631, 1953.
24. Brehmer, Anderson E.: Diagnostic importance of punch biopsy in zoster and simplex. *Acta. Dermat.* (Stockholm) **45**:267-71, 1965.
25. Brezak, S.: Clinical evaluation of a treatment for removal of pedal warts. *JAPA,* **44**:43-44, 1954.
26. Brody, B.: A method of treatment of recurrent verruca. *JAPA,* **51**:416-417, 1961.
27. Brown, J. B. and Fryer, M. D.: Repair of surface defects of the foot; resurfacing foot by plastic surgery for defects such as plantars and traumatic thermal and radiation lesions. *JAMA,* **146**:628, 1951.
28. Bunney, M. H., et al: Treatment of plantar warts at home. A critical appraisal of new preparation. *Practioner,* **207**:197-204, 1971.
29. Bunney, M. H., et al: Molluscum contagiosum of the sole. A rare diagnosis of a rare condition? *Brit. J. Derm.,* **81**:623-625, 1969.
30. Buske, E.: Injection therapy for verruca. *J. Nat. Assoc. Chir.,* June, 1947.
31. Buske, E. G.: Local parenteral and oral bismuth therapy for verrucae. *JAPA,* **53**:269-271, 1963.
32. Carpenter, W. E.: Results of a 4-year study of injection therapy in the treatment of plantar warts. *JAPA,* **51**:407-409, 1961.
33. Carslow, R. W. and Neill, J.: Linseed oil in the treatment of plantar warts. *Brit. J. Derm.,* **75**:280-284, 1963.
34. Carter, R. T.: Verruca, some impressions from a study of 118 cases. *JAPA,* **59**:336-339, 1969.
35. Cherup, N., et al: Treatment of plantar warts with ultrasound. *Arch. Phys. Med. Rehab.,* **44**:602-604, 1963.
36. Church, R.: Virus infections of skin. *Practitioner,* **192**:629-638, 1964.
37. Ciuffo, G.: Innesto positivo con filtrato di verruca volgare. *G. Ital. Mal. Venereol.,* **48**:12, 1907.
38. Clark, G. H.: The charming of warts. *J. Invest. Derm.,* **45**:15-21, 1965.
39. Cohen, E. L.: Inefficancy of sodium bismuth triglycollamate in the treatment of warts. *Brit. J. Derm.,* **70**:254-255, 1958.
40. Conway, H., Hugo, N. E., and Tulenko, J. F.: *Surgery of Tumors of the Skin,* 2nd ed., Thomas, Springfield, Ill., 1966.
41. Cramer, L. L.: A new injectable agent in plantar wart therapy. *J. Nat. Assoc. Chir.,* **42**, #3, 1952.
42. Cramer, L. L.: Parenzyme injection for plantar warts. *JAPA,* **48**:526-528, 1958.

43. Crow, K. D. and Scott, O. L. S.: Treatment of plantar warts with carbon dioxide snow. *Lancet,* **2**:312-314, 1954.
44. Demeur, E. W.: Treatment of verruca by the intradermal method. *Clin. J. Chir. Pedic. Surg.,* Sept., 1937.
45. Desforges, J. A.: Mosiac and mutiple plantar verrucae. *J. Nat. Assoc. Chir.,* **46**:699-700, 1956.
46. Dingman, R. O. and Grabb, W. C.: The intractable plantar wart. *J. Mich. Med. Soc.,* **62**:296-299, 1962.
47. Dollin, J.: Aureomycin therapy of multiple verrucae. *N.Y. State Med. J.* **50**:705, 1950.
48. Dorland, W. A. N.: *The American Illustrated Medical Dictionary,* Saunders, Phila., 1952.
49. Dorsey, C.: Liquid nitrogen therapy of warts. An evaluation. *Calif. Med.* **98**:33-34, 1963.
50. Dugan, H. E.: Low-dose roentgen therapy of verrucae plantaris. *Arch. Derm.,* **90**:202-204, 1964.
51. DuVries, H. L.: New approach to the treatment of intractable verruca plantaris. *J. Nat. Assoc. Chir.,* **44**:26-36, 1954.
52. Ecker, H. A.: The use of Salisacom as pre-op preparation for excision and flap repair of plantar warts. *Plast. Reconstr. Surg.,* **37**:461-463, 1966.
53. Eden, T.: Elimination of Weight-bearing as Verruca Therapy. Lecture at *N.Y. State Podiatry Conv.,* March, 1952.
54. Eilard, U., et al: Herpes simplex; A statistical and clinical investigation based on 669 patients. *Dermatologia* (Basal) **130**:101-106, 1965.
55. Epstein, W. L. and et al: Viral antigens in human epidermal tumors: Localization of an antigen to moluscum contagiosum. *J. Invest. Derm.,* **40**:51-59, 1963.
56. Epstein, W. L. and Kligman, A. M.: Treatment of warts with cantharidin. *Arch. Derm.,* **77**:508-511, 1958.
57. Falknor, G. W.: Molluscum contagiosum of the foot: A clinical note. *JAPA,* **59**:482, 1969.
58. Fitzpatrick, et al: *Dermatology in General Medicine,* McGraw-Hill, Inc., 1971.
59. Gardner, L. W., et al: Bone destruction of a distal phalanx by periungual warts. *Arch. Derm.,* **107**:275-276, 1973.
60. Genner, J.: Location of wart virus antigen in human plantar warts. *Acta, Derm. Vener.,* **51**:361-364, 1972.
61. Giannini, J. T.: Digital shortening procedure for complicated plantar warts. *Plast. Reconstr. Surg.,* **13**:130, 1954.
62. Gibbs, R. C.: Differential diagnosis of plantar verrucae. *JAPA,* **59**:90-92, 1969.
63. Gilbert, R. S. and Williams, M. J.: Local injection of Vitamin A (Keramin) for plantar verrucae. *U.S. Armed Forced Med. J.* **10**(7):843-847, 1959.
64. Goldschmidt, H. and Kligman, A. M.: Experimental innoculation of humans with ectodermotropic viruses. *J. Invest. Derm.,* **31**:175-182.
65. Goldsmith, W. N.: *Recent Advances in Dermatology,* Churchill, London, 1936.
66. Goodman, J. M.: Liquid nitrogen therapy of warts and other skin lesions. *Canad. Med. Assoc. J.,* **82**:628-630, 1960.
67. Goodman, L. S. and Gilman, A.: *The Pharmacological Basis of Therapeutics,* 4th ed., MacMillan, London, 1970.
68. Grady, E. D.: A simple method of removing plantar warts. *G.P.,* **25**:89, 1962.

69. Greeley, P. W.: Plastic repair of radiation ulcers of the sole. *U.S. Nav. Med. Bull.,* **45**:827, 1945.
70. Grigg, W. K. and Wilhelm, G.: Epidemiological study of plantar warts among school children. *Pub. Health Rep.,* **68**:985-988, 1953.
71. Hemlich, H. A.: Mosiac verrucae. *J. Nat Assoc. Chir.,* **42**:27-28, 1952.
72. Henao, M. and Freeman, R. G.: Inflammatory molluscum contagiosum. *Arch. Derm.,* **90**:479, 1964.
73. Henenfeld, M.: Verruca plantaris. A differential diagnosis. *JAPA.,* **50**:453-461, 1960.
74. Hertz, C.: as cited in *Modern Foot Therapy.* Gross, R. H., Modern Foot Therapy Publ. Co., N.Y., pp. 240-242.
75. Hollander, L. and Hardy, S. M.: Failure of aureomycin therapy in warts. *Arch. Derm. Syph.,* **62**:714-715, 1950.
76. Horwitz, O. and Marker, T.: The efficiency of electrocaustic, keratolytic and placebo treatment in patients with single warts. *Acta. Derm. Vener.,* **40**:127-134, 1960.
77. Hutchinson, R.: Treatment of warts by viral interference, *Practitioner,* **204**:700-704, 1970.
78. Hyman, D.: Plantar warts, newer treatments. *N.Y.J. Med.,* **63**:1680-1681, 1963.
79. Ignatoff, W. B.: Verruca therapy. *J. Nat. Assoc. Chir.,* **44**:37-47, 1954.
80. Juel, Jensen B. E.: The Natural History of Shingles, *Jour. R. Coll. Gen. Pract.,* **20**:323-327, 1970.
81. Jurgensen, W. W. and Peartree, S. P.: The plantar wart: Treatment with radiation therapy. *Miss. Vall. Med. J.,* **79**:288-289, 1957.
82. Kanoor, P.: Primary herpes simples infection of fingers in nurses, *Dermatologia (Basel)* **134**:346-350, 1967.
83. Katz, J.: Bloodless surgical technique for verruca plantaris, *J. Nat. Assoc. Chir.,* **38**:31-32, 1948.
84. Kingland, H. D.: Cryotherapy in the treatment of verrucae. *JAPA.,* **52**:435, 1962.
85. Klauder, J. V.: Treatment of some dermatoses by local injection of Vitamin A., *Arch. Derm.,* **81**:253-259, 1960.
86. Kurtin, A. and Yontef, R.: Podophyllum therapy of warts. *Arch. Derm. Syph.,* **57**:395, 1948.
87. Lal, S., et al: Herpes zoster. *J. Assoc. Physicians India,* **18**:853-854, October, 1970.
88. Lapidus, P. W.: Orthopedic skin lesions of the soles and toes. *Clin. Orth.,* **45**:87-100, 1966.
89. Laurie: Plantar warts, *Brit. Med. J.,* **3**:116-118, 1972.
90. Lawrence, K. R.: Treatment of verrucae with smallpox vaccine. *JAPA.,* **61**:12-19, 1971.
91. Lehman, R. A. and Manning, M. M.: Treatment of plantar warts by local injection of Vitamin A. *Clin. Med.,* **6**:1153, 1959.
92. Lerner, L. H.: Management of plantar verrucae via excision and curettage. *JAPA.,* **49**:11-14, 1959.
93. Lever, W. F.: *Histopathology of the Skin,* 4th ed., Lippincott, Phila., 1967.
94. Levy, A. E.: Treatment of plantar warts with radiation. *W. Va. Med. J.,* **54** (12):474-475, 1958.
95. Lieberman, H.: An empirical treatment for mosiac verrucae. *JAPA.,* **50**:737, 1960.
96. LoCricchio, J. and Haserick, J. R.: Hot-water treatment for warts. *Cleve. Clin. Quart.,* **29**:156-161, 1962.

97. Lutzner, M. A.: Molluscum contagiosum, verruca and zoster viruses. *Arch. Derm.,* **87**:436-444, 1963.
98. Lyell, A. and Miles, J. A. R.: The myrmecia. A study of inclusion bodies in warts. *Brit. Med. J.,***1**:912-915, 1951.
99. Lynch, F. W. and Karon, I. M.: Formaldehyde. *Arch. Derm. Syph.,***62**:803-813, 1950.
100. Manilla, G. T., et al: Treatment of plantar warts. *Rocky Mt. Med. J.,* **62**:42, 1965.
101. Marples, M. J.: *The Ecology of the Human Skin,* Thomas, Springfield, Ill., 1965.
102. Marshall, J.: *Diseases of the Skin,* Livingston, Edinburgh, 1960.
103. Marten, R. H.: "Plantar Warts", in *Modern Treatment Yearbook,* 1962, pp. 215-221.
104. Massing, A. M. and Epstein, W. L.: Natural history of warts. *Arch. Derm.,* **87**:306, 1963.
105. Matthewson, J. B.: Liquid nitrogen in dermatology; successful method of treating plantar warts. *N.Y. J. Med.,* **55**:374-375, 1955.
106. May, H.: Surgical treatment of intractable plantar warts. *Surg. Clin. N. Amer.,* **31**:607-616, 1951.
107. McDowell, F.: Plantar warts, plantar calluses and such. *Plast. Reconstr. Surg.,* **51**:196-197, 1973.
108. McGee, A. R.: Apparent antagonism of vaccinia and wart virus. *Cancer,* **20**:1647, 1967.
109. McGee, A. R.: Wart treatment by vaccination with smallpox vaccine. *Canad. Med. Assoc. J.,* **99**:119-121, 1968.
110. McLaughlin, C. R.: Plantar warts: A plea for rational treatment. *Lancet,* **1**:168-169, 1948.
111. McQuire, C. P.: Role of the plantar flap in the surgical treatment of plantar warts. *J.S. Carolina Med. Assoc.,* **58**:483-484, 1962.
112. Mendelson, C. G. and Kligman, A. M.: Isolation of wart virus in tissue culture. Successful reinoculation into humans. *Arch. Derm.,* **83**:559-562, 1961.
113. Monroe, C. W.: Plantar warts. *Plast. Reconstr. Surg.,* **17**:168-183, 1956.
114. Montgomery, A. H.: Classification and X-ray therapy of verruca plantaris. *J. Nat. Assoc. Chir.,* April 1929.
115. Montgomery, A. H. and Montgomery, R. M.: Roentgen ray therapy of plantar warts, *N.Y. State J. Med.,* **63**:1532, 1963.
116. Montgomery, R. M.: Dermatological care of the painful foot. *J.B.J.S.* (Amer.), **46**:1129-1136, 1964.
117. Montgomery, R. M.: Painful cutaneous lesions of the feet. *Southern Med. J.,* **63**:615-519, 1970.
118. Murphy, J. C., et al: Chloroquine treatment of warts. *Rocky Mt. Med. J.,* **62**:25-26, 1965.
119. Noyes, W. F.: Structure of human wart virus, *Virology,* **23**:65-72, 1964.
120. Ogilvie, M. M.: Antibody to human wart virus. *J. Hyg. Camb.,* **68**:479, 1970.
121. Ormond, C. S.: Combined use of formaldehyde and bismuth tartrate in treating verrucae. *J. Nat. Assoc. Chir.,* **42**:31-34, 1952.
122. Ormond, C. S.: Review of injection therapy in treating plantar verrucae. *J. Nat. Assoc. Chir.,* **46**:455-457, 1956.
123. Overcast, V. C.: Curetting verrucae with minimum hemorrhage. *J. Nat. Assoc. Chir.,* **47**:187-188, 1957.

124. Pass, F., et al: Antigens of human wart tissue. *J. Invest. Derm.,* **56**:305-310, 1971.
125. Pass, F. and Marcus, D. M.: Wart-associated antigens I and II. *J. Invest. Derm.,* **60**:301-311, 1973.
126. Peck, S. and Ignatoff, W. B.: Verruca therapy. *J. Nat. Assoc. Chir.,* **44**:37-47, 1954.
127. Perlstein, S. M.: The treatment of viral verruca. *Antibio. Med.,* **5** (3):186-188, 1958.
128. Perreira-Marques, J.: Considerations and treatment of plantar warts by hypertonic occlusive strapping. *Clin. Med.,* **72**:795-802, 1965.
129. Perry, G. M.: Molluscum contagiosum. A case report. *JAPA,* **54**:32-33, 1964.
130. Postelthwaite, R.: Antiviral activity in extracts from lesions of molluscum contagiosum. *Virology,* **22**:508-517, 1964.
131. Prazak, G. and Lazar, M. P.: Periungual warts. *Arch. Derm.,* **69**:230, 1954.
132. Prazak, G. and Thomas, D. E.: Curettage treatment of plantar warts. *Arch. Derm.,* **74**:204-205, 1956.
133. Prose, P. H., et al: Molluscum contagiosum virus in adult human skin cultures. An electron microscopic study. *Amer. J. Path.,* **55**:349-366, 1969.
134. Purgett, D. L.: Radiology in chiropody. *J. Nat. Assoc. Chir.,* **40**:29-38, 1950.
135. Pyrhonen, S. and Pentlinen, K.: Wart-virus antibodies and the prognosis of wart disease. *Lancet,* **2**:1330-1332, 1972.
136. Reeves, R. J. and Jackson, M. T.: Roentgen therapy of plantar warts. *Am. J. Roentg.,* **76** (5):977-978, 1956.
137. Robbins, S. L.: *Pathology,* 3rd ed., Saunders, Phila., 1969.
138. Robinson, D. W.: Treatment of complications of plantar warts (repair by skin grafts). *Arch. Surg.,* **66**:434-439, 1953.
139. Rook, A., Wilkinson, D. S., and Eibling, F. J. G.: *Textbook of Dermatology,* Davis, Phila., 1968, pg. 753.
140. Rowe, R. J. and Gray, J. M.: Ultrasound therapy of plantar warts. *Arch. Derm.,* **82**:1008-1009, 1960.
141. Rowe, R. J. and Gray, J. M.: Ultrasound therapy of plantar warts. *Arch Phys. Med.,* **46**:273-274, 1965.
142. Rubin, D., et al: Muscle paralysis in herpes zoster. *Calif. Med.* **103**:261-266, October, 1965.
143. Rulison, R. H.: Warts: A statistical study of 921 cases. *Arch. Derm.,* **46**:66, 1942.
144. Sakurane, Y. and Sugan T.: Treatment of verruca plana juvenalis with gamma globulin. *Arch. Derm.,* **82**:640-1, 1960.
145. Samitz, M. H. and Dana, A. S.: *Cutaneous Lesions of the Lower Extremities,* Lippincott, Phila., 1971, pp. 50-53.
146. Sauer, G. C.: *Manual of Skin Diseases,* 2nd ed., Lippincott, Phila., 1966, pp. 222-251.
147. Schenkman, S. P.: Curettage and cautery of verrucae. *JAPA,* **51**:658, 1961.
148. Shellow, H.: Treatment of verruca by local injections of bismuth. *Ill. Med. J.,* **66**:932, 1934.
149. Shields, C. et al: Plantar warts. *Brit. Med. J.,* **3**:170, 1972.

150. Silverman, L. J.: Rationale of a treatment for mosiac verruca based on the local adaptation syndrome. *JAPA,* **55**:522-526, 1965.
151. Smiler, I.: Surgical galvanism for warts. *JAPA,* **58**:225-228, 1968.
152. Stankler, L.: A critical assessment of the cure of warts by suggestion. *Practitioner,* **198**:690-694, 1967.
153. Steinberg, M. D.: A new treatment for resistant warts. *Surgery,* **39**: 642, 1956.
154. Stern, J.: Quinocaine injection therapy for verrucae. *JAPA,* **51**:413-415, 1961.
155. Suppan, R. J. and Besterman, G.: Curettage and chemotherapy for verrucae. *JAPA,* **53**:265-286, 1963.
156. Surman, O. S., et al: Hypnosis in the treatment of warts. *Arch. Gen. Psych.,* **28**:439-441, 1973.
157. Sutton, J. S. and Burnett, J. W.: Ultrastructure changes in dermal and epidermal cells of skin infected with molluscum contagiosum virus. *J. Ultrastruc. Research,* **26**:177-196, 1969.
158. Taub, J. and Steinberg, M. D.: Porokeratosis plantaris discreta, a previously unrecognized dermatopathological entity. *Intl. J. Derm.,* **9**:83-90, 1970.
159. Tenzel, J. H. and Taylor, R. L.: An evaluation of hypnosis and suggestion treatment for warts. *Psychosomatics,* **710**:252-257, 1969.
160. Thompson, K. W.: Treatment of verrucae with smallpox vaccine. *JAMA,* **207**:368, 1969.
161. Thomson, J. G. and Rauschkolbt, J. E.: Contact X-ray treatment of the common wart. *Arch. Derm. Syph.,* **65**:553-556, 1952.
162. Thomson, S.: Formalin treatment of plantar warts. *Brit. J. Derm.,* **55**:267, 1943.
163. Thomson, S. and Coles, R. B., et al: Treatment of warts with formaldedhyde and nobecutane. *Practitioner,* **194**:378-381, 1965.
164. Twain, M.: *Tom Sawyer.*
165. VanGasse, J. J. and Miller, R. F.: Epidemiologic study of plantar warts. *Arch. Ped.,* **75**:279-284, 1958.
166. Vaughn, D. T.: Direct vs. underwater method in treatment of plantar warts with ultrasound. *Phys. Ther.,* **53**:396-397, 1973.
167. Vickers, C. F. H.: Plantar warts. *Brit. Med. J.,* **2**:743, 1961.
168. Walter, E. L., Jr., et al: Localization of specific antigen in human warts. *Arch. Path.,* **79**:419-423, 1965.
169. Walz, D. U.: Podophyllum for plantar warts. *Arch. Derm.,* **65**:490, 1952.
170. Weinstock, B. S.: An evaluation of the curettage treatment of plantar verrucae. *J. Nat. Assoc. Chir.,* **47**:67-68, 1957.
171. Wile, V. J. and Kingery, L. B.: Etiology of common warts; a preliminary report of an experimental study. *JAMA,* **73**:970-973, 1919.
172. Woolf, W. H.: Capillary tube acid applicator for verrucae. *JAPA,* **49**:18-20, 1959.
173. Woolf, W. H.: Verruca; its possible relationship to other neoplasms. *JAPA,* **52**:893-898, 1962.
174. Wygant, L. A.: Hypnosis in a case of multiple verrucae. *JAPA,* **51**:660, 1961.
175. Zichichi, D.: Molluscum contagiosum: A case report. *JAPA,* **59**:274-275, 1969.

SECTION III

HYPERKERATOTIC LESIONS AND RELATED SKIN GROWTHS

Introduction

The words hyperkeratosis, keratoma, keratodermia, callous, and tyloma are often synonymous with the term keratosis. They all are employed to signify some form of thickening of the outer layer of the epidermis. Therefore, the term keratosis may be employed for any solitary discrete palmar or plantar keratotic lesion, a collection of localized palmar or plantar thickenings, or for any diffuse palmar or plantar thickening. Actually hyperkeratosis encompasses the category of corn and calluses which have often been wrongly referred to as keratoses. Calluses represent a mild inflammatory response of the body to longstanding, intermittent or continuous friction or pressure which is confined to certain predisposed areas of the skin. These areas are seen most frequently on the palms and soles. It is in these locations that the skin undergoes shearing or frictional forces over an underlying bone to induce callus formation. It is for this reason that callus formation is present in many biomechanical abnormalities of the lower extremity. An area which is receiving a pathologic amount of weight-bearing will tend to develop callus due to the change in pressure or friction to that area. The so-called pinch callus located on the medial surface of the hallux toe develops due to a combination of a short first metatarsal bone with limitation of motion at the metatarsophalangeal joint, and pinching of the skin of the medial aspect of the hallux due to abnormal pressure exerted by the shoe. If a metatarsal head becomes hypertrophied or an abnormal parabola of the metatarsals exists, intractable plantar keratoma might occur. Other biomechanical abnormalities such as hammertoes, hallux valgus deformity, or other changes in bone structures cause callus formation due to structural change creating additional pressure and friction.

The keratoses of the palms and soles refer to, and are associated with, a group of uncommon, ordinarily hereditary, and otherwise idiopathic disorders. They are characterized by histologically indistinguishable thickening of the epidermis, and have a predilection for the palms and soles.

There are some keratoses found on other parts of the body that

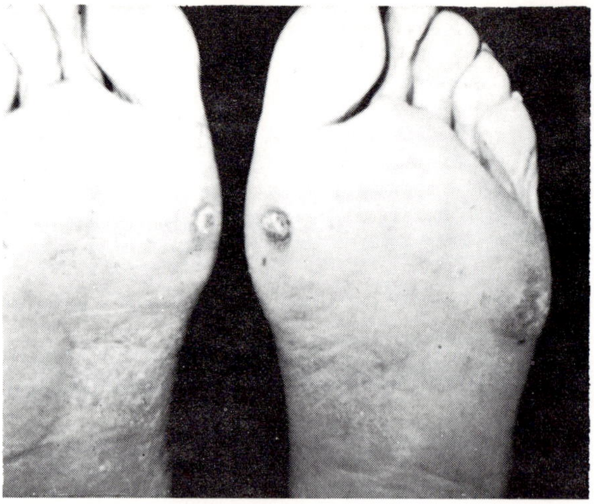

FIGURE 3-1

Common Plantar Callouses due to biomechanical changes in foot structure. Such lesions may also run in families or specific foot types.

are often induced by sunlight, such as actinic or senile keratoses. Some also develop in association with internal disorders such as the internal malignancies seen with acanthosis nigricans and the keratosis associated with syphilis and carcinoma of the esophagus. An uncovering of significant internal diseases is important, for cutaneous keratosis may be an invaluable clue to certain internal abnormalities.

There are many precancerous keratoses which, by definition, refer to those conditions having a tendency toward malignancy. Some of these are arsenical keratoses, occupational keratoses, solar keratoses, senile keratoses, and cutaneous horn.

It is for this reason that a thorough history of the lesion be taken when a patient presents with a keratotic abnormality. The history itself may disclose the cause of the lesion; for instance, in cases where there has been chronic arsenic ingestion earlier in life or a past history of over treatment with roentgen rays for a plantar verrucae. The history may give clues to the etiology of the lesions. It is obvious that a keratosis is not of the idiopathic type from this type of information. Also, a complete occupational and sports history may resolve an unexplainable keratotic lesion for a frictional or traumatic etiology and may distinguish it from the idiopathic keratosis.

In this subsequent chapter we will attempt to discuss some of the keratotic lesions of the foot and to correlate them with the differences in etiology, sites of predilection, incidence, onset, and treatment.

In order to do this, the lesions are categorized into hereditary idiopathic keratosis, and precancerous keratoses.

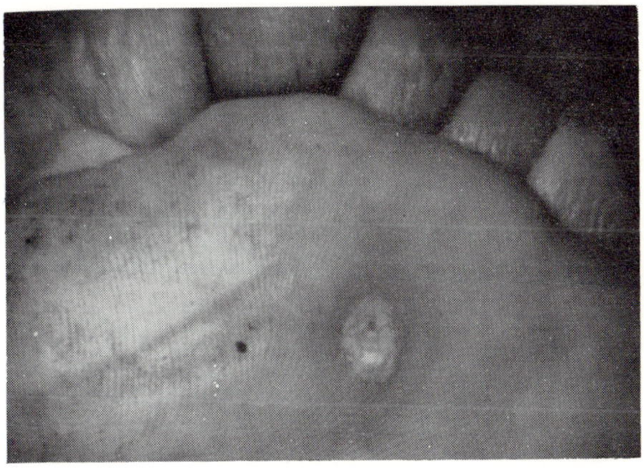

FIGURE 3-2

Painful keratoma with involvement of the third metatarsal head. These lesions are often confused with plantar warts.

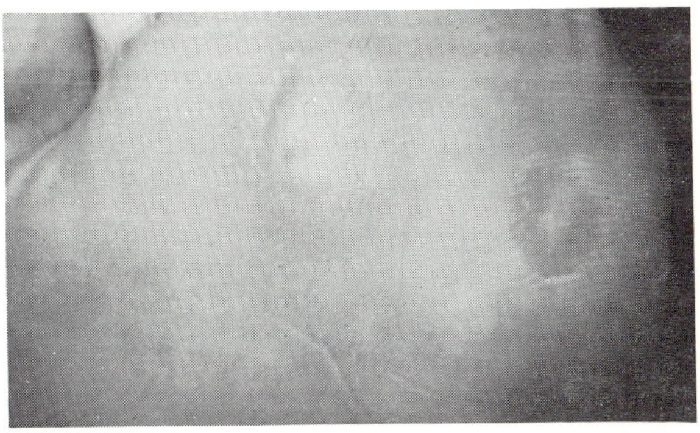

FIGURE 3-3

Painful keratoma under second metatarsal head with associated plantar fibrosis. This is typical of "Morton's Syndrome" characteristics.

TABLE I
CHART SUMMARY

DISEASE	ETIOLOGY	ONSET	SITE OF PREDILECTION
Keratosis palmaris et Plantaris Hereditaria (Unna Thost)	Hereditary	Early in life (3-12 mo.)	Palms and soles
Keratosis Punctata	Hereditary	First decade insidious	Confined to palms and soles.
Keratosis Striata	Hereditary	First few weeks of life	Palms and soles, buttock, elbow, axillae and knee.
Mal de Meleda	Hereditary (Recessive)	First two years of life	Palms and soles with ichthyotic changes elsewhere on body.
Papillon-LeFevre Syndrome	Hereditary	First 6 mo. of life	Palms and soles periodontal changes.
Arsenical Keratosis	Prolonged absorption of arsenicals.	Usually later in life	Palms and soles and generalized throughout body.
Occupational Keratosis	Exposure to chemical substances	Few weeks after exposure	Palms and soles especially arms and hands.
Senile Keratosis	Increased exposure to sunlight	Usually later in life.	Exposed parts - face, ears, scalp, hands, forearms, and neck.
Cutaneous horn	Actual cause not known	Later decade of life	Scalp, forehead, nose, hands, and feet.
Keratoacanthoma	Over-exposure to sunlight, tars, petroleum	Solitary lesion sixth decade, Multiple lesions early in life.	Middle of face, dorsum of fore-arm, and hands

ASSOCIATED FINDINGS	TREATMENT
Fissuring of the skin	Keratolytics highly resistant to treatment
Hyperhidrosis, rarely	Keratolytics; Removal of keratotic plugs.
Ocular, mucous membrane and nail changes.	Similar KPPH
Local hyperhidrosis usually present	Unsatisfactory; Keratolytics and oral vitamin A.
Psoriasiform patches, ectopic calcification of dural membranes	Similar for KPPH Dental consultation
Circumscribed edema, esp. of lower eyelids, alopecia, reticulated hyperpigmentation and onychorrhexis.	Withdraw source of arsenic exposure, destroy keratosis or epitheliomas.
Dermatitis, malignant changes, ulcerations	Prophylactic procedures (mild soothing ointments), hygenic working conditions, excision of residual ulcers
Malignant degeneration	Local destructive measures (electrocoagulation cautery), biopsy if excised.
Transition into malignancies	Electrodesication, radium and roentgen rays, carbon dioxide snow.
	If lesion does not resolve spontaneously within a 4-6 week period, surgical excision.

Idiopathic Hereditary Keratosis

1. KERATOSIS PALMARIS ET PLANTARIS HEREDITARIA (KPPH)

History

KPPH was first described by Thost in 1880, under the name of congenital ichthyosis of the palms and soles.[23] Toward the end of the 19th century, Paul Unna differentiated this condition described by Thost from ordinary calluses which were clinically very similar to KPPH.[32] Unna emphasized the hereditary factors in KPPH and noted that the condition was not traumatically induced as in calluses. He named this former condition Keratoma Hereditarium Palmaris et Plantaris by which the condition is still frequently remembered. It was accepted as Unna-Thost Disease in honor of these two pioneer observers.

Definition

The disease is congenital or inherited as an autosomal dominant, symmetrical, diffuse cornification of the horny layer of the epidermis of the palms and soles. This condition is not rare and involves both sexes equally. It is widespread in the white or yellow races, but uncommon in the negro.

Onset

KPPH manifests itself early in life. Some babies destined to have the defect, appear normal at birth, but in others, the skin of the palms and soles may be redder than normal and scaling appears at the end of the first week.[68] In most instances however, the first noticeable change is a thickening of the skin, which becomes apparent between the age of 3 to 12 months, or exceptionally later and has frequent association with hyperhidrosis. The hyperkeratosis increases gradually and usually reaches its full development in the second decade or early adult life.

Clinical Picture

The thickening involves all of the palms and soles and the flexor surfaces of the fingers and toes. The change from the

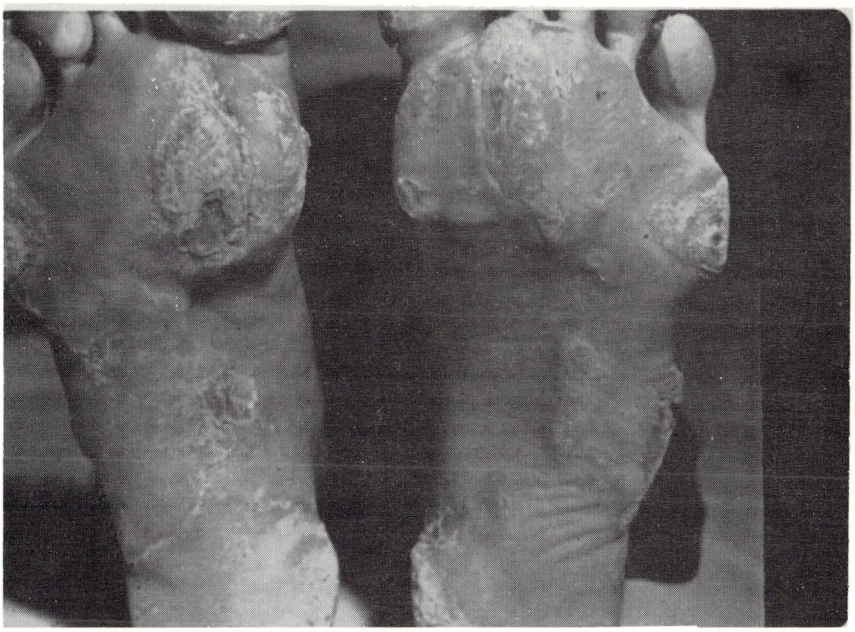

FIGURE 3-4

Diffuse and irregular plantar hyperkeratosis: Discoloration is often due to hyperhidrosis. (Courtesy W. V. R. Shellow, M.D., Los Angeles, California)

keratotic to the normal skin is sometimes marked by a narrow, red line. On the soles, the weight bearing areas are more severely affected, while the skin beneath the arch is relatively normal.

The thickness of the hornified layer of the palms and soles varies from several millimeters to a centimeter. Its surface may be smooth, uneven, porous, pitted, or verrucous. In the young, the affected parts are white and waxy, or translucent; later in life they become opaque and yellowish-brown or almost black in color.

The palms and soles may be rubbery in consistency or covered by thick, firm or rigid plates. There is fissuring of the unyielding skin, especially on the palms. The cracks may occur either on the normal furrows or independent of them, producing a mosaic-like effect. The fissures often involve the corium and cause considerable tenderness and pain, especially if they become inflammed. A variable amount of scaling is present, and it is usually more abundant in the winter. The nails may remain normal or become thick, opaque, and malformed. In some cases, the hyperkeratosis may be limited to either the soles or the palms.

Treatment

The condition is highly resistant to treatment. The skin may, however, be made more flexible and pliant by the use of plasters, ointments, keratolytics, and topical steroids. Therapy must be carried on indefinitely. Perhaps the most important aspect of treatment is continuous debridement of the hyperkeratotic tissues. This in itself will help render a patient asymptomatic.

2. KERATOSIS PUNCTATA

History

Keratosis punctata was first described in a mentally retarded epileptic Hindu by Davies — Colley in 1879. He referred to this condition as a disseminated clavus of the hands.[24] Although an

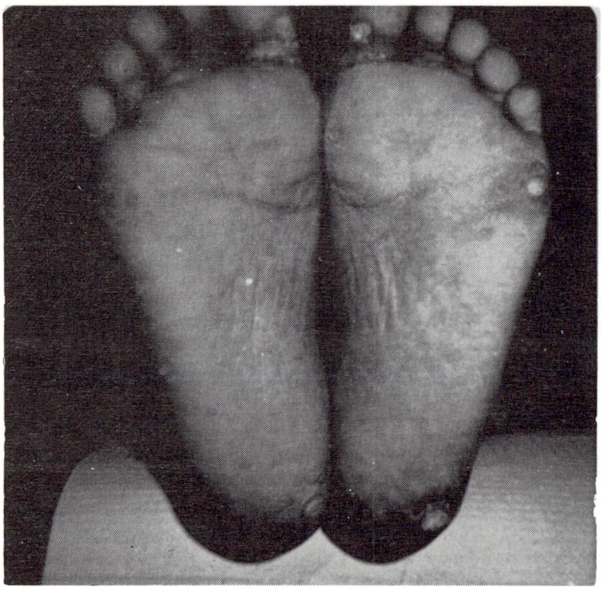

FIGURE 3-5

Severe and painful isolated keratotic lesions of unknown etiology and diagnosis. Hand lesions revealed keratosis at several of the phalangeal joint areas.

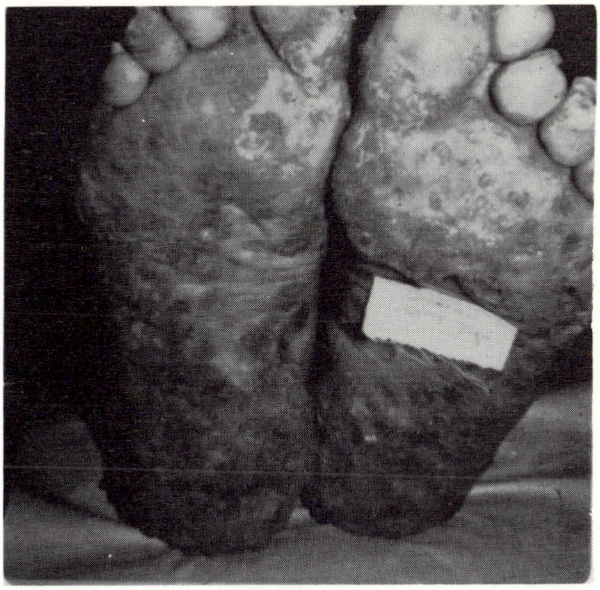

FIGURE 3-6

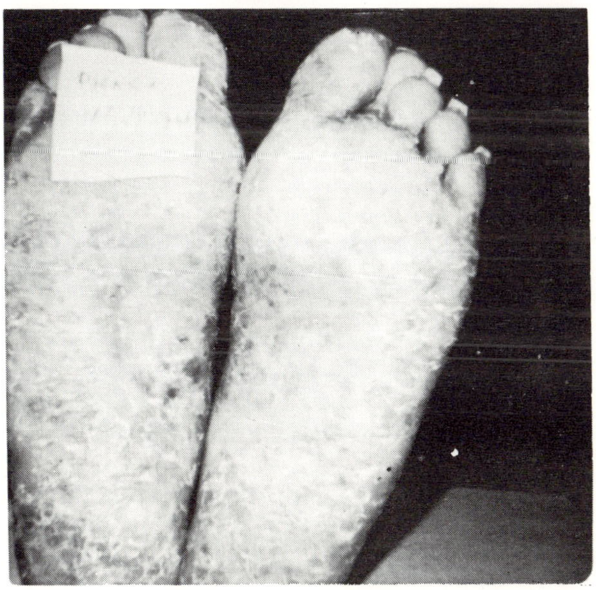

FIGURE 3-7

Hereditary Keratosis Palmaris et Plantaris. Treatment consisted of constant debridement and a multitude of associated treatment and results from 12 months of therapy.

original description of the conditon has also been attributed to Besnier, Hallopeau, and Claisse, there is little tangible evidence to support such claims.[16]

Definition

Keratosis punctata is an inherited autosomal dominant and manifests as a congenital defect of cornification, with the development of scattered discrete, warty papules on the palms and soles. The disease is rather rare and it is distributed equally between the two sexes. There does not appear to be a racial predilection in Europe, although most of the reported cases in the United States are negroes.[32]

Onset

The condition usually makes its appearance insidiously, shortly after puberty, although the onset may occur during adult life or be postponed as late as the fifth decade.

Clinical Picture

A few to several hundred or more lesions are distributed symmetrically on the palms or soles or both. The palmar aspects of the fingers and the plantar surfaces of the toes are also involved. There is some predilection for areas subject to pressure, with the center of the palm and the long arch being less frequently invaded.

The lesions are usually imbedded in the skin; however, some may be elevated as much as 1.0 cm above the skin. They are characterized by multiple, discrete, yellow to dark-bronze shiny, firm and round, and/or polygonal conical keratotic papules varying from 1.0 mm to 1.0 cm or more in size. There is no tendency to coalescence or spontaneous shedding of the lesion. The skin between the horny papules remains normal in all aspects. In extreme cases, the numerous horny masses create a pavement-like appearance on the palms and soles. In spite of their numbers, the papules cause no subjective symptoms, except in rare instances following hard labor, walking, or the direct application of pressure. Hyperhidrosis is not often an associated finding, but it does occur occasionally.

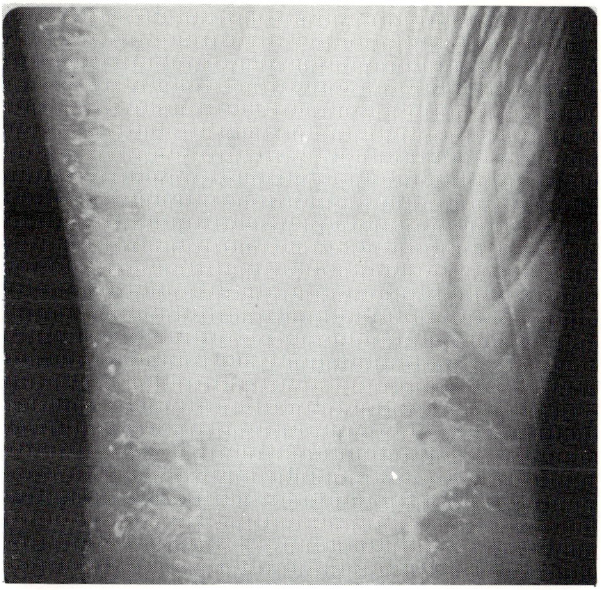

FIGURE 3-8

Punctate forms of keratosis. Commonly referred to as seed corns.

Differential Diagnosis

Keratosis punctata may be distinguished by its familiar occurrence — well circumscribed keratotic papules and crateriform pits, normal intervening skin, and limitation to the palms and soles. It is most frequently confused with arsenical keratosis and papular syphilis. The disease must also be differentiated from warts, keratosis follicularis, porokeratosis of Mibelli, angiokeratoma, lichen planus, and psoriasis.

Treatment

There is no satisfactory treatment for this condition. Once established, it usually remains for life. General palliative care is usually a measure of limiting it. Therapy is essentially the same as for KPPH. Pain may be relieved in some instances by removal of the central inverted triangular keratotic plugs, which usually leave a shallow depressed center.

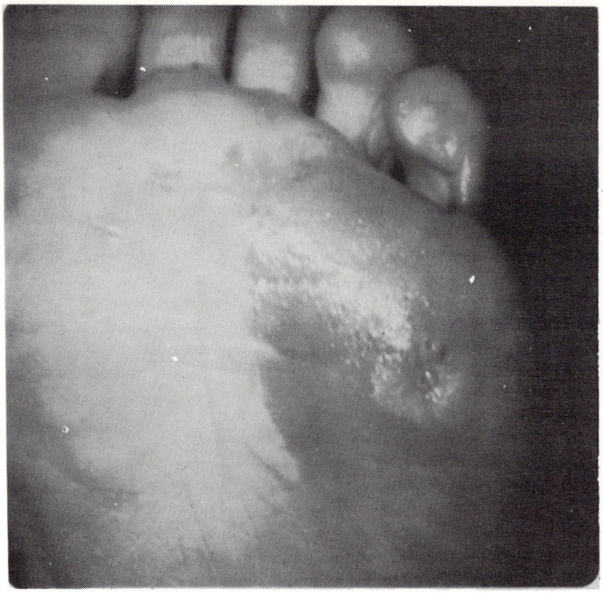

FIGURE 3-9

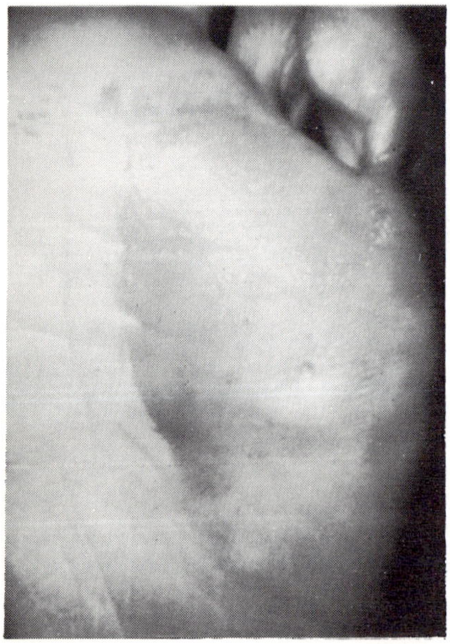

FIGURE 3-10

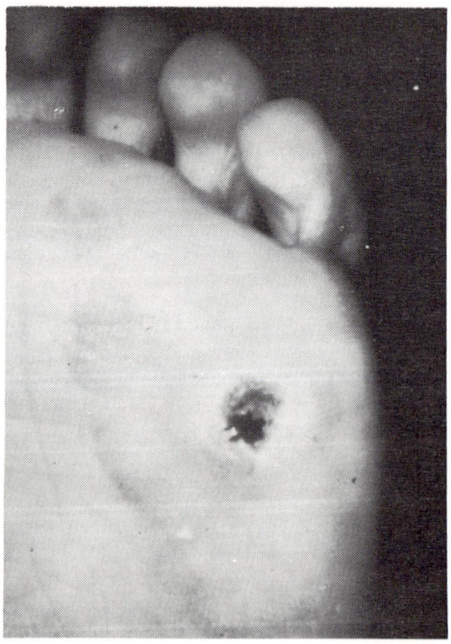

FIGURE 3-11

Isolated seed corn. Excision of plantar lesion with blunt currettement often results in a cure.

3. KERATOSIS STRIATA

History

There have been two specific varieties of striate palmar keratoses that have been described: the first, without other abnormalities in keratinization was described first by Siemens in 1929; the second, associated with other abnormalities of keratinization, was described in the 1920's by Gassman, Riehl, Bruhauer, and Fuhs.[91] The type described by these latter authors, also referred to as keratosis multiformis by Siemens, is remarkably similar to pachyonychia congenita.[32] Both conditions are congenital and associated with a multitude of disorders such as: nails, mucous membrane, and occular abnormalities. These are also seen with either generalized ichthyotic lesions or follicular keratosis in addition to the striate keratosis. Common locations for these associated keratosis are the buttocks, elbows, and axillae.

Clinical Picture

Clinically, keratosis palmo-plantaris striata lies between KPPH and keratosis punctata. Although the clinical manifestations vary greatly, the lesions are usually confluent keratotic plaques, but do not involve the entire palmar and/or plantar surfaces. The abnormality derives its name from the fact that in the affected families, there is a tendency for palmar thickenings to take on a linear arrangement. This configuration is usually less evident on the soles.

It is usually associated with keratotic lesions elsewhere except when it is a manifestation of ichthyosis hystrix, nevus unius lateris, or epidermal nevus. Not all individuals in the same family follow the characteristic pattern. In some, there are icthyosis hystrix-like thickenings of the palmar aspects of the fingers in conjunction with diffuse hyperkeratosis of the palms. In others, involvement may vary from one or two small thick patches on the palms to complete marked hyperkeratosis of the palms and soles. A frequent manifestation in this group is hyperkeratosis of the extensor surfaces of the knees and thickening along the sides of the achilles tendon.

Onset

Keratosis striata is transmitted as an autosomal dominant. Although the condition has been reported to have an onset within the first few weeks of life, as well as in teenagers, it usually is discovered within the first few years of life, generally somewhat later than KPPH. It persists throughout life with exacerbations during the winter time due to the occurrence of fissures.

Treatment

This disease can be ameliorated by similar measures recommended for KPPH, such as: palliative care and softening ointments and plasters of salicylic acid, etc.

4. MAL DE MELEDA

History

Mal de Meleda was first described by Stulli in 1826,[47] when he reported 11 cases. Haverka subsequently viewed this condition as Hansen's Disease, but in 1898, Neumann disproved this concept.[19]

Definition

It is a congenital symmetrical cornification of the palms and soles associated with ichthyotic changes elsewhere on the skin. It occurs endemically on the Island of Meleda, which is in the Adriatic, off the coast of Yugoslavia.

Etiology

Unknown. It is believed to be inherited in a recessive manner.

Onset

Typically, the disease appears within the first two years of life, usually at about the sixth month. The first manifestation is redness of the palms and soles which is soon followed by roughening and thickness. Eventually the palms and soles become covered by a thick horny layer surrounded by a bluish zone about 1.0 cm wide. Characteristically, it is associated with keratotic lesions on the dorsum of the fingers and toes, wrists, ankles, elbows, and knees.

Clinical Picture

The clinical picture varies from thick yellowish, translucent, and waxy hyperkeratosis to a dense brown or black horny plate with many fissures. Local hyperhidrosis is usually present. It is questionable as to whether it deserves a special classification from diffuse keratosis palmaris et plantaris. This is a very rare condition.

Treatment

Treatment is unsatisfactory and mainly consists of applications containing salicylic acid. Temporary improvement has been reported after 300,000 units of Vitamin A daily.[47] Topical urea 20-40% has also been utilized.

5. PAPILLON — LEFEVRE SYNDROME

History

Hyperkeratosis palmo-plantaris and premature periodontoclasia is the name originally given by Papillon and LeFevre in 1924 to a disease then considered to be Mal de Meleda with dental abnormalities, where the deciduous teeth usually have fallen out because of periodontitis by five years of age. The same process occurs with the permanent teeth so that by 16 years of age, the patient is endentulous. Later it was recognized as an independent entity, possibly even related to KPPH. About thirty cases have been described to date.[10] This syndrome has been considered a recessive form of Unna-Thost disease; however, this relationship is speculative. The condition is inherited as a recessive trait, both sexes being equally susceptible.

Onset

The syndrome begins in the first six months of life.

Clinical Picture

The mild hyperkeratosis that develops is restricted to the palms, whereas the keratosis that develops on the soles extends to contiguous areas. Erythema precedes the keratosis and ceases during the peridontal changes that occur. The keratosis is scaly on the periphery and usually associated with bromhidrosis. Aside from the palmar-plantar hyperkeratosis and periodontal changes, other characteristics are present with this syndrome such as psoriasiform patches on the extremities, or ectopic calcification of the dural membranes.[10]

Treatment

Therapy is similar to that employed for KPPH.[22] Dental consultation is also necessary for treatment of the oral manifestations.

Pre-Cancerous Keratosis

1. ARSENICAL KERATOSIS

Definition

The continued absorption of arsenical compounds either as drugs or in the course of certain occupations, may produce hyperkeratosis on the palms and soles.

History

The arsenical keratoses of the palms and soles are one of the most common manifestations of chronic arsenical intoxication. They were probably first recognized by Henoch and Romberg in 1851.[64]

Clinical Picture

The keratoses are usually found on the soles; however, if present on the palms, usually the grip areas are most commonly affected. This type of lesion can also be seen affecting the sides of the digits and can be generalized throughout any area of the body. They may be induced by prolonged ingestion of inorganic arsenic. Usually the unexposed areas are more involved. Often cutaneous changes that may occur with chronic arsenical intoxication include circumscribed edema, especially around the lower eyelids, alopecia, and reticulated hyperpigmentation.[14] Ungual changes consisting of onychorrhexis may occur.

Onset

The first objective evidence of impending keratoses, usually following local symptoms of pruritis and erythema, is the occurrence of various-sized discrete, flattened, amber colored, keratotic papules. Following this, the involved regions become infiltrated with punctate keratoses. The skin of the palms and soles take on a leathery appearance which is due to hyperhidrosis. A certain number of arsenical keratoses may degenerate into squamous cell carcinoma after long latent periods. Neubauer

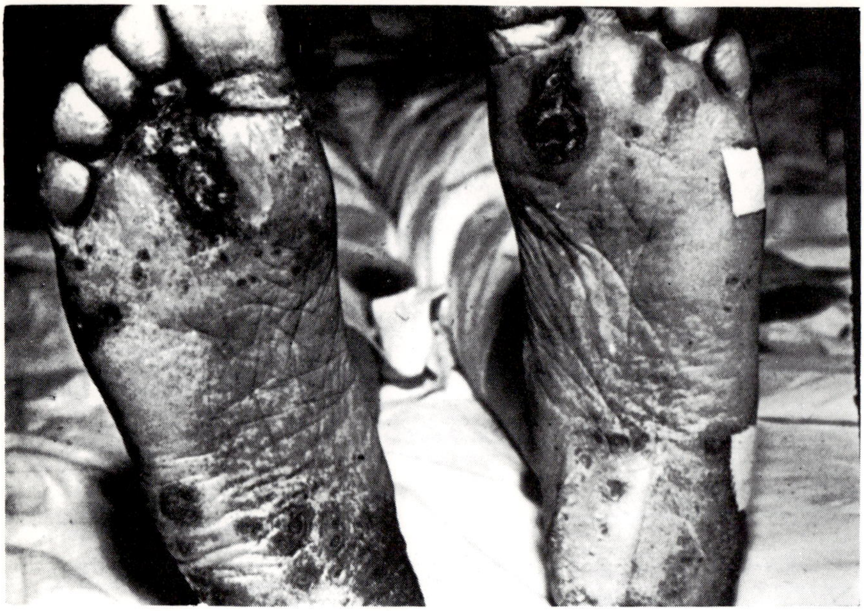

FIGURE 3-12

Arsenical Keratosis. This results from exposure to industrial, medicinal or environmental sources of arsenic. (Courtesy of William V. R. Shellow, M.D., Los Angeles, California)

reported 116 epitheliomas preceded by keratoses out of 143 cases.[64] Cutaneous arsenical intoxication is very often associated with internal neoplasms. Reports by Sommers and McMann in 1953 investigated this association in a study of 27 patients.[93] Significantly higher incidences of lung cancer, visceral cancer and carcinoma of the cervix were found to be present amongst those exposed to arsenic in one form or another, than those not exposed.[82] The particularly dangerous arsenical keratosis is the lesion that is located at the muco-cutaneous junction. Patients should be warned against repeated absorption of certain arsenicals. Bowen's disease may also be frequently seen.

Differential Diagnosis

Arsenical keratoses are to be differentiated from keratosis punctata and those conditions simulating it. It may also resemble late secondary syphilis. On the sole, epitheliomatous degenera-

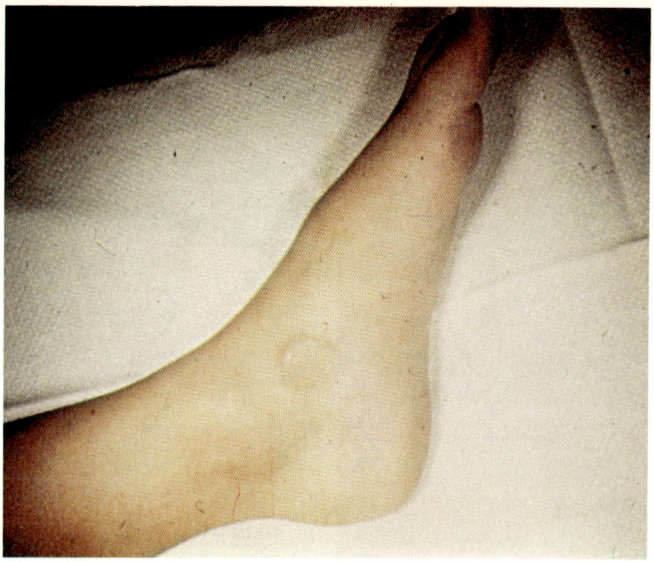

Granuloma Annulare — Ring like lesions which are often several lesions. Vary from flesh color to pale red nodules. Usually are asymptomatic and often resolve after several years. (Courtesy of Isadore Zeligman, M.D., Baltimore, Maryland.)

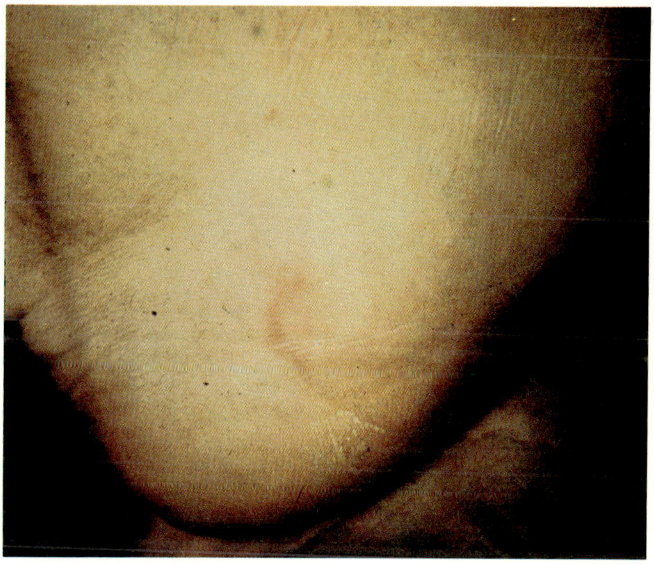

Larva Migrans — ("Creeping Erruption") Early cutaneous lesions involving the heel. Most common symptom is pruritis. (Courtesy of William V. R. Shellow, M.D., Los Angeles, California)

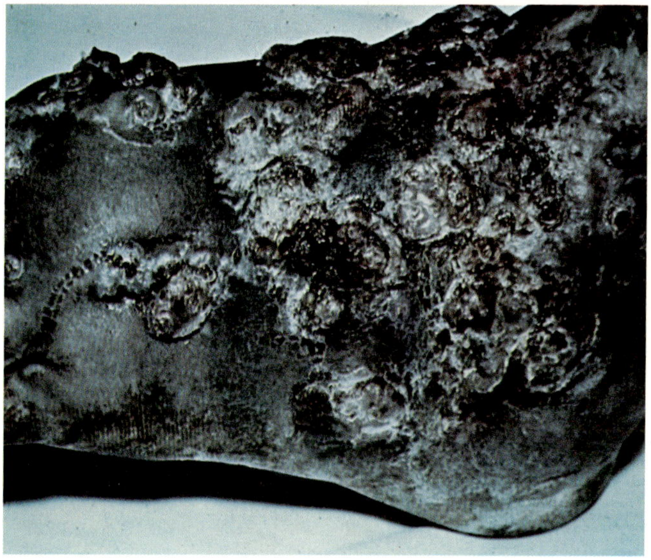

Mycetoma (Madura Foot) — This is a chronic infectious disease of the subcutaneous tissue, skin, and bone, characteristically of the foot, usually following trauma. Etiology: Actinomyces, Nocardia, Streptomyces, Madurella, Allescheria and Phialophora species. (Courtesy of William V. R. Shellow, M.D., Los Angeles, California.)

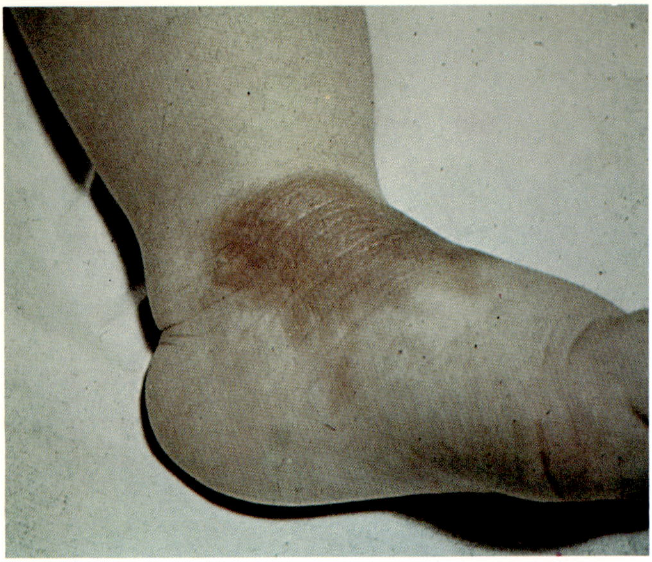

Solitary Mastocytoma — The isolated mastocytoma is usually a reddish-brown oval plaque or nodule noted at or soon after birth. These spontaneously involute within a few years without incidence of associated systemic disease. (Courtesy of William V.R. Shellow M.D., Los Angeles, California.)

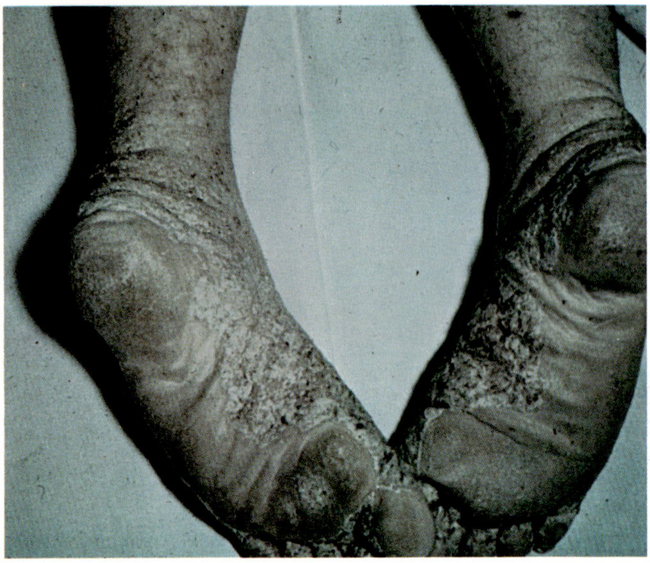

Norwegian Scabies — Characterized by overwhelming number of mites leading to extensive hyperkeratosis and crusting of the palms, soles, limbs, scalp and trunk. Differential diagnosis — psoriasis. (Courtesy William V.R. Shellow, M.D., Los Angeles, California.)

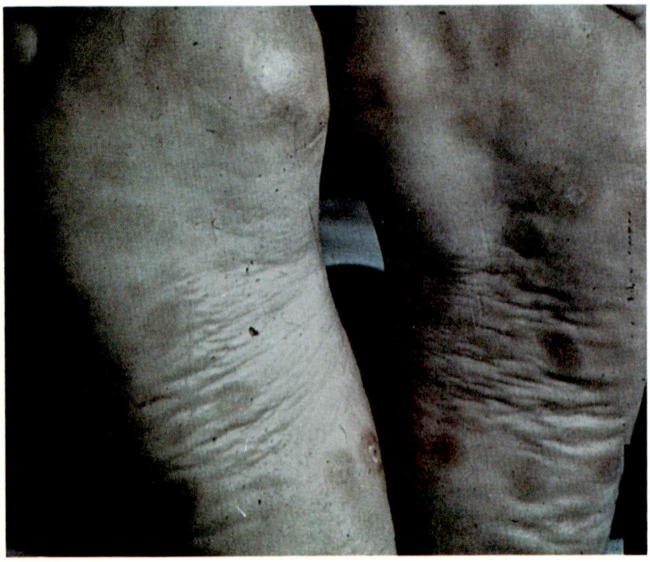

Secondary Syphilis — Characteristic plantar lesions. (Courtesy William V.R. Shellow, M.D., Los Angeles, California.)

tion of an arsenic keratosis may produce a lesion suggestive of malum perforans. Any suspicious precancerous keratosis should be biopsied, for a microscopic examination can usually distinguish between the various keratoses and will always confirm transformation from a benign state to a malignant one.[78]

Treatment

The best therapy for arsenical keratosis is to prevent the source of arsenical exposure if possible, and locally, to destroy the existing keratosis or epitheliomas. Probably the use of any destructive modality such as electrodessication, curretage, chemocautery, the administration of superficial X-rays or grenz-ray, and the application of solid carbon dioxide snow and liquid nitrogen may be employed. Vitamin A administration has also been reported to be effective.[41]

2. OCCUPATIONAL KERATOSIS

Definition

In addition to arsenicals, other chemical substances may produce dermatoses such as chronic inflammatory conditions or hyperkeratoses, from which carcinomas occasionally arise. Many occupations provide periodic exposure of their workers to these etiologic agents. Other agents such as tar, various products of coal distillation, mineral oil and its derivatives, hydrocarbon components and related substances such as pitch, creosote, asphalt, anilines, anilmache, and shale oils, rarely cause keratosis. They more commonly cause contact dermatitis and, less frequently, skin cancer. Occupational keratoses occur with the exposure to berryllium and silicon asbestos, and a hyperkeratotic palmar eruption in nurses and physicians can be due to contact with streptomycin, as well as to atabrine in solvents.

Onset

Gradual onset with continuous exposure.

Clinical Picture

A great number of workers are exposed to these substances, and their dangerous influence assumes an important role in industrial and social medicine.[27] Individuals who handle paraformaldehyde, an agent used extensively in industry, may develop yellow-brown hyperkeratoses of the flexor aspects of the hands, as well as the feet. Paraffin workers may also develop palmar keratoses.[105] Habitual contact with hydrocarbon occurs among many categories of workers such as tar distillers, fisherman, roofers, lampblack workers, chimney sweepers and gas works employees.

The frequent forerunner of the malignant changes is usually a keratoses or acute dermatitis which may become chronic when the patient continues to be exposed to the above mentioned substances. Many years, however, may elapse before a carcinoma develops in the damaged skin.[27] The lesions are located mainly on the arms and hands where the skin is most exposed to the irritant, or they are found at the sites where additional irritation, such as friction by the clothes and profuse perspiration, influences the skin.

In paraffin carcinoma, the preceding dermatitis is often noticed within a few weeks after exposure. If the exposure is continued, a hyperplastic eczematoid dermatitis with wart-like hyperkeratoses may develop, which frequently undergoes malignant transformation after several years. In contrast, tar carcinoma may occasionally develop without any visible previous alteration of the skin.

Treatment

The therapy in occupational precanceroses consists chiefly of prophylactic procedures, hygienic working conditions and timely discontinuance of contact with the offending substances as soon as the first sign of cutaneous irritation appears. (Symptomatic treatment with mild, soothing ointments usually leads to complete healing of irritated skin). The residual keratoses, or ulcers that refuse to heal after change of occupation should be biopsied or destroyed with electrosurgery. Treatment administered early enough may prevent cancer development.

3. ACTINIC KERATOSIS (SENILE OR SOLAR KERATOSIS)

Definition

Actinic keratosis is so commonly associated with senile atrophy of the skin that it may be considered part of the syndrome. The etiologic factors are certainly the same in both lesions.

Onset

These lesions are common in caucasoids. The areas most commonly affected are the exposed parts such as the face, ears, bald scalp, and hands and, less frequently, the forearms and neck. It is seldom seen on the foot; however it may appear on the posterior aspect of the foot where there has been exposure to the sun and rarely, if ever, on the plantar surfaces. This condition is especially common in farmers, cattlemen, and sailors. This is because senile keratoses are more prevalent in regions receiving a great deal of sunshine, and their incidence is higher in rural than in urban districts.[97] They are more common in fair-skinned persons. The negro, whose pigment and heavy layer protects against the sun's rays, is rarely affected by actinic keratoses or malignant cutaneous epithelioma.

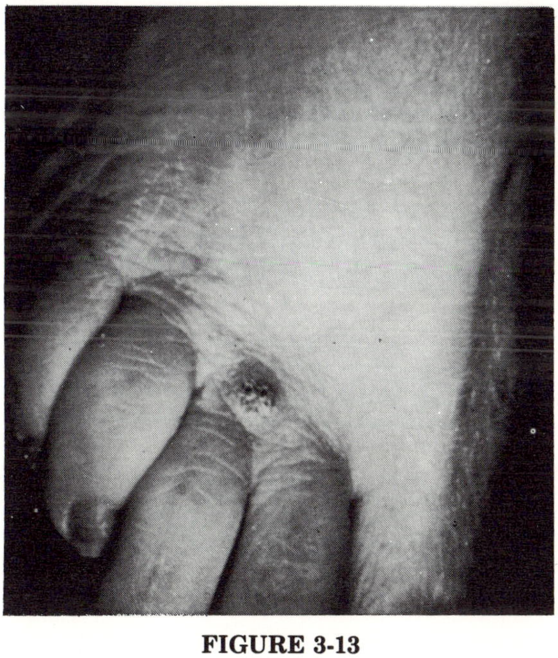

FIGURE 3-13

Actinic Keratosis. Commonly referred to as solar or senile keratosis. (Courtesy Richard Gibbs, M.D., New York City, New York)

Squamous cell carcinoma may develop from actinic keratoses; it may be seen on the hand and rarely on the foot. The possibility of metastasis of a squamous cell carcinoma from actinic keratosis can occur, but is infrequent. Bowen's disease has also been observed. If the lesion shows signs of growth, has an indurate border, or has begun to ulcerate, biopsy from a small excised tissue wedge should be performed.

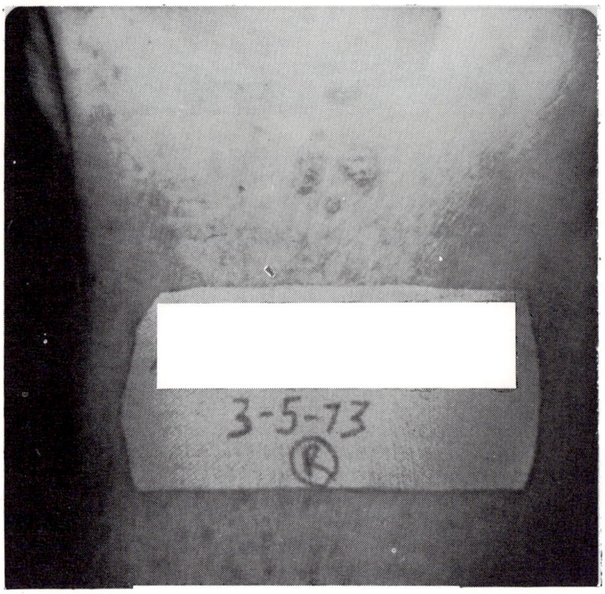

FIGURE 3-14

Seborrheic Keratosis of the dorsal aspect of the foot.

Treatment

In the treatment of this condition, early diagnosis and proper treatment are essential factors in the prevention of skin carcinoma. Senile keratosis without infiltration, ulceration, or inflammation can be cured by local destructive measures. This may be done with electrocoagulation, or excision. Another method employed is with the use of cryotherapy ($C0_2$ Snow, liquid nitrogen). Keratoses may also be removed by the application of an acid such as trichloracetic. Topical 5-flourouracil is now the treatment of choice for multiple lesions.

4. CUTANEOUS HORN

Definition

Cutaneous Horn is defined as a papillary, medullated, horny growth seated on a circumscribed, warty base. The cutaneous horns are rare, but the term cornu cutaneum is also commonly applied to various non-medullated keratotic growths, which are comparatively common.[98]

Onset

This hypertrophic skin lesion is encountered most frequently in the later decades of life, but is seen occasionally in children. It may arise from a sebaceous cyst, wart or scar, but more frequently originates from a keratosis. The actual cause is not known.

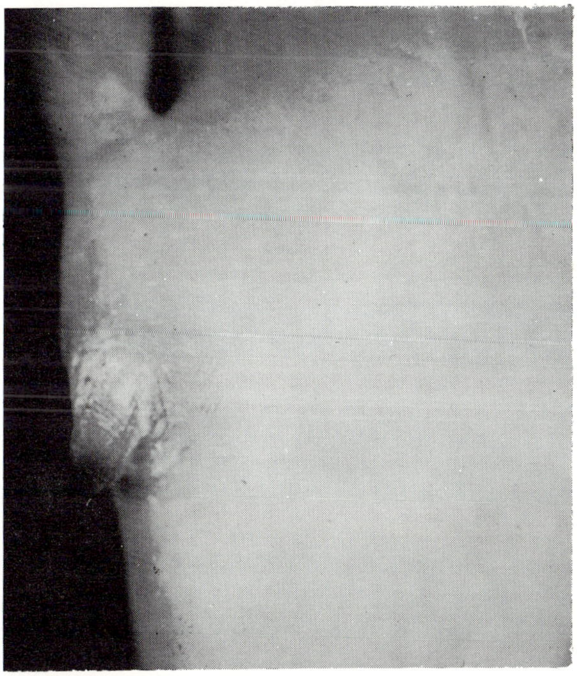

FIGURE 3-15

Cutaneous Horn on the sole. These horn shaped lesions may develop with persistant hyperkeratotic development and whether they are true cutaneous horns is questionable. (Courtesy Jeffrey Yale, D.P.M., Ansonia, Connecticut)

Clinical Picture

The sites of predilection are the scalp, the forehead, the nose, the hands and the feet, and less frequently on the penis, scrotum, and buttocks.

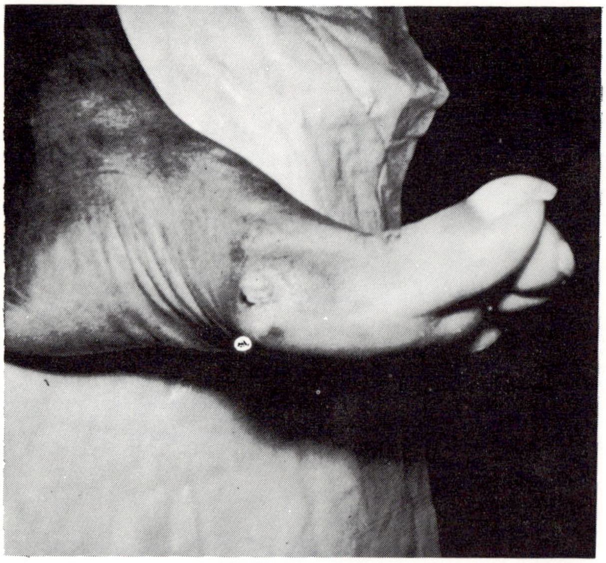

FIGURE 3-16

Cutaneous Horn over first metatarsal joint.

The lesions are solid, dry, conical, outgrowths, variable in size and shape. They may be straight or curved, round, oval, or irregular. They are usually a normal skin color, but may be yellowish, brownish, or blackish. Their bases are concave or flattened and often verrucous. The greater part of the lesion is composed of keratin.[57] These are considered in the category of precancerous lesions because a certain percentage of cutaneous horns become cancerous. Squamous cell carcinoma, basal cell carcinoma, and actinic keratosis have been seen at the base of the cutaneous horn. Lobert estimates that about 12% will make this transition. It usually occurs at the base of the horn, and usually after the age of forty.[57]

Histologic Picture

True cutaneous horns always have one or more hypertrophied papillae for a base. The intrapapilliary vessels are greatly increased in size. The interior of this horn consists of columns of anuclear corneous cells, arranged in folded laminae, the interspaces being filled with horny wedges and homogenous appearing masses of corneous substance.[98] Approaching malignant change is indicated by a broken basal cell layer, dyskeratosis, atypical epithelial proliferation and inflammation.

Treatment

The treatment of choice is excision,[32] however, electrodessication is often used.

5. KERATOACANTHOMA

Definition

Keratoacanthoma is generally a firm, raised nodule with a central crater. It is not a pre-malignant lesion, but it is often confused with squamous cell carcinoma.

History

This condition was first described in the late nineteenth century by Jonathan Hutchinson, who reported a crateriform ulcer of the face.[78]

Onset

The greatest incidence of solitary lesions is in the sixth decade; whereas multiple lesions appear earlier in life. The most common location for the keratoacanthoma is the middle of the face, although the dorsum of the forearm or hand is frequently involved. There have been few reports of palmar and plantar lesions. These were reported by Rook and Moffatt, Rabut and Hewitt, and Levy.[55,79,94] The lesions on the palms and soles are sometimes not unlike keratosis punctata; whereas such a diagnosis would not be considered in the typical, centrally depressed lesion found elsewhere. Other conditions to consider are verrucae vulgaris and those diseases simulating keratosis punctata. However, the rapid onset of the lesions is highly suggestive of keratoacanthoma. Multiple lesions should be watched.

Clinical Picture

The lesion presents itself as a solitary, dome-shaped nodule with a depressed, keratin filled center. When the lesion disappears spontaneously it may leave no trace, or a barely visible scar. The multiple variety is much more likely to disappear spontaneously. The lesion or lesions of keratoacanthoma are rarely, if ever, seen in blacks, and are usually found in caucasians who have had overexposure to sunlight or to tars and petroleum. These tumors have been considered pre-malignant lesions, but rarely become malignant. They closely resemble the histological picture of squamous cell carcinoma, grade one.

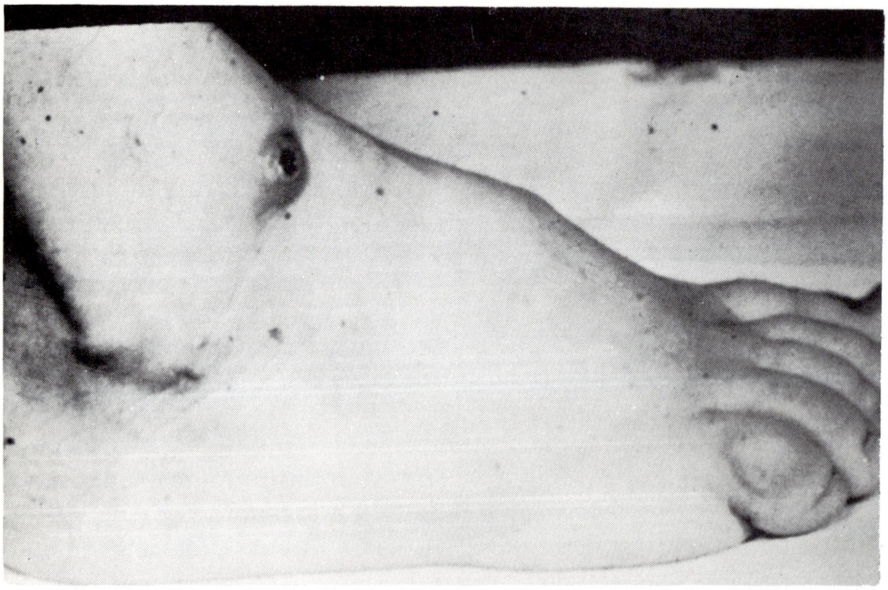

FIGURE 3-17

Keratoacanthoma: These lesions may closely resemble squamous cell carcinoma both clinically and histologically. (Courtesy James Ganley, D.P.M., Norristown, Pennsylvania)

Treatment

The fully developed tumor requires only four to six weeks for its maturation. After a stationary period of several months, the nodule usually resolves within a few weeks.[78] It is debatable whether or not the lesions should be treated surgically, even though adequate excision usually presents a cure.

Cutaneous Lesions and Manifestations of Systemic Disease

There are many dermatologic lesions that may appear as tumors and there are many systemic diseases which have a tendency to affect the pedal skin. This monograph will not attempt to list all the various conditions, however, it was thought appropriate that some of the common systemic diseases seen in the podiatry offices as well as rare manifestations which are seldom seen, be mentioned.

1. KERATOSIS ASSOCIATED WITH INTERNAL MALIGNANCIES — ACANTHOSIS NIGRICANS

History

This disease was first described by Sigmond Pollizer and Janousky in 1890.[28,74] Acanthosis nigricans or Acanthosis keratosis is a dermatosis of remarkably uniform appearance. The disease is quite rare, as only 400 malignant cases have been recorded since Pollitzer, in collaboration with Paul Unna, published the first case.[74]

Definition

Acanthosis nigricans may be a chronic inflammatory disease which in adult life may be associated with cancer of some internal organ.

Onset

The mode of onset is variable and the cutaneous lesions may develop slowly and insidiously, or rapidly.

Clinical Picture

The significant elements of the gross skin changes are a characteristic, symmetrical distribution, soft velvety papillary hypertrophy, hyperpigmentation, and hyperkeratosis. The most common sites of predilection are the axillae, the nape of the neck, the genitals, the inner thighs, the elbow bends, the umbilicus, the perianal region may also be involved where the dorsal aspect of the hands and feet are uncommon findings. In some cases the lips, the anterior neck, the areolae of the nipples, and large areas of the trunk may be affected and mucous membranes are only occasionally involved.

The earliest manifestations are usually pigmentary in character, the affected skin assuming a reddish, brownish, or blackish hue which gradually fades off in the margin of the lesions. The epidermis becomes thickened, but without accompanying induration, and the natural lines of the skin are exaggerated. These changes are followed by the development of numerous soft, millet-seed to pea-sized papillary growths. Hyperkeratosis of the palms and soles is a common finding. The color of the lesion may vary from gray, slate, or yellow to all shades of brown and black. Within the hyperpigmented areas, depigmented areas are frequently present and this is due to inflammation. The hair is usually destroyed in the affected areas and the nail bed may be pigmented and the nail plate longitudinally grooved.

Types

There are generally three forms. Curth in 1966 revealed each type was classical of a separate disease.[28]

1. Malignant adult form — which is always associated with cancer, usually of an internal organ. The malignant refers to the association with malignancy, not to a malignant course of the dermatosis itself.
2. The juvenile form — which is inherited and benign.
3. Pseudo-acanthosis nigricans — is probably due to simple obesity and is undoubtedly an environmentally induced disorder simulating the genetic type.

Many cases of acanthosis nigricans occur in patients with cancer. Ninety-two percent of these malignancies were found in the abdominal viscera, mostly in the stomach, and almost all of the abdominal cancers had abdominal metastases.

Treatment

The treatment of this disease is at best symptomatic unless regression occurs after extirpalation of the malignancy. The prognosis of juvenile acanthosis nigricans as a dermatosis is that of an incurable, though in itself not a dangerous anomaly, comparable to a widespread nevus. However, the prognosis of the juvenile benign variety is good but often darkened by the association of a systemic disease. If it develops after the age of forty, it is almost certain to be indicative of cancer.[58] In this case, exploratory laparotomy should be done because of the probability of metastases.

2. ARTHRITIC DISEASES

Gouty Arthritis

Gouty arthritis is a metabolic disease characterized by a marked elevation of blood uric acid. The clinical picture of gout is usually that of a rapid onset of pain, redness, and swelling around

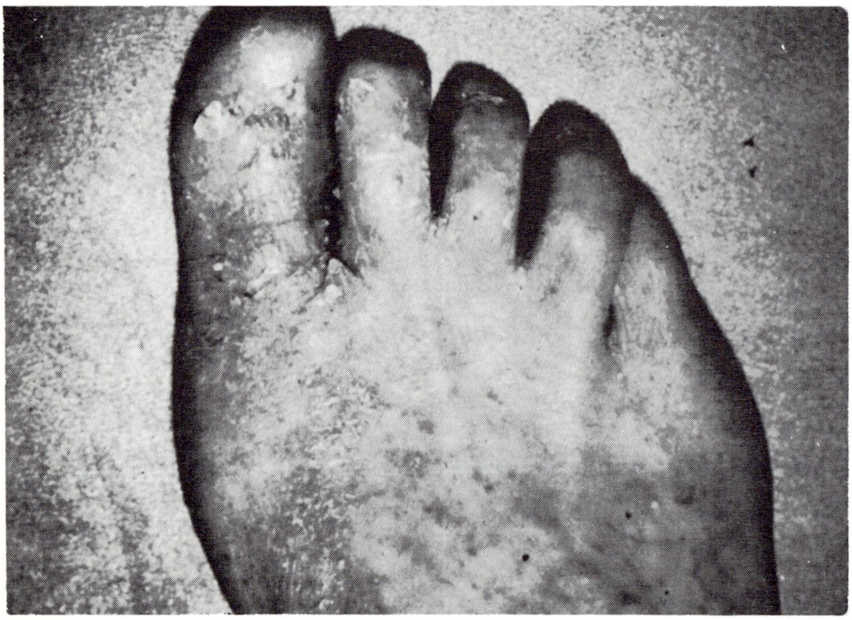

FIGURE 3-18

Dyskeratosis Congenita: This is a rare, often fatal genodermatosis characterized by reticulated hyperpigmentation, atrophic changes of the dorsal aspect of the hands and feet, loss of nails, leukokeratosis of the mucous membranes, and hyperkeratosis of the palms and soles. (Courtesy W. V. R. Shellow, M.D., Los Angeles, California)

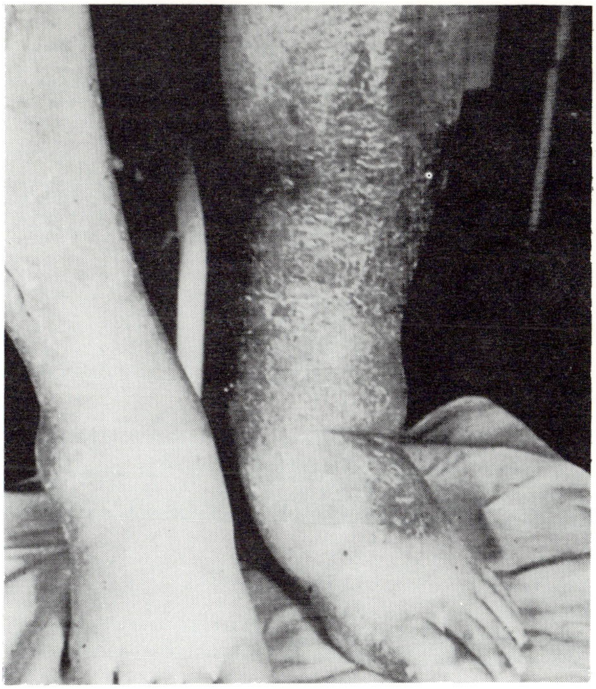

FIGURE 3-19

Elephantiasis Nostras Verrucosa: Chronic lymphatic blockage, sometimes due to recurrent erysipelas; can lead to verrucous changes in the skin. (Courtesy William V. R. Shellow, M.D., Los Angeles, California)

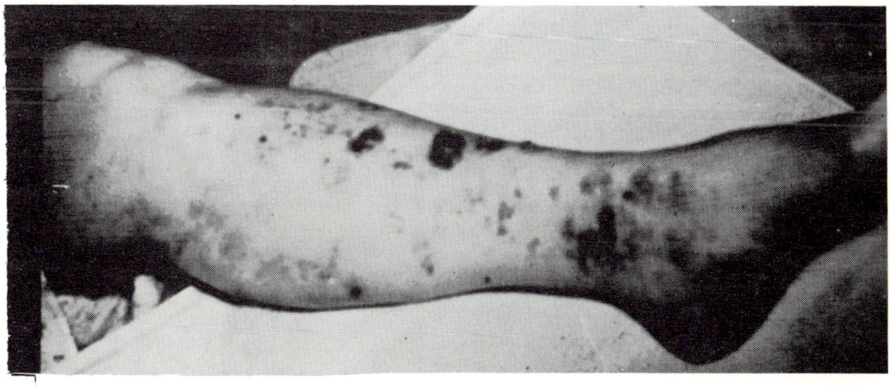

FIGURE 3-20

Angiokeratoma — Dark pigmented areas with hyperkeratosis or warty appearance. The Mibelli form is seen in the lower extremities. (Courtesy James Ganley, D.P.M., Norristown, Pennsylvania)

the joint, particularly the first metatarsophalangeal joint of the foot. Individuals who have had gouty arthritis for many years usually develop uric acid crystals around or within the joint. These uric acid crystals may form to such degree that lesions may be noticeable on clinical inspection of the foot. These gouty lesions caused by deposition of uric acid crystals may become very irritating, particulary on pressure from shoes.

Treatment

The treatment of gout consists of numerous drugs, primarily those which increase the amount of uric acid excretion from the body. However, in those lesions which may be present in gouty arthritis from uric acid crystal formations, surgical excision of such gouty tophi may be necessary in order to render symptomatic relief. However, these lesions may recur due to further deposition of uric acid salts.

Osteoarthritis

This is a non-inflammatory form of arthritis which usually results from wear and tear of the joint cartilage whether it be due to age, trauma, or other types of joint responses. The joints which seem to be the most commonly involved along with the fingers, however, are the weight-bearing joints of the foot.

Signs and Symptoms

Affected individuals usually have stiffening of the joints particularly in the early mornings and again late in the evenings after rest. The joints may also show some signs of swelling. These swellings are known as Heberden's nodes. They may develop as small little firm, nodular, asymptomatic lesions around joints.

Diagnosis

Diagnosis of these lesions and the condition is usually not difficult and a careful history is most often the clue to one's diagnosis.

Treatment

The treatment is usually that of symptomatic care, including aspirin and rest of the affected parts.

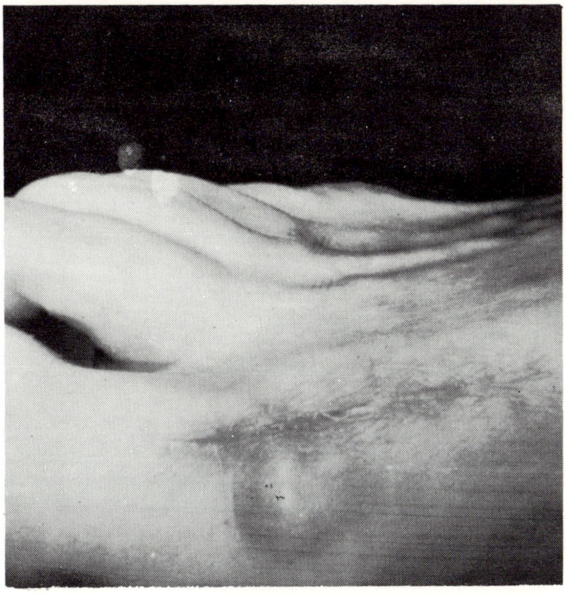

FIGURE 3-21

Rheumatoid Nodule: Lesion developed post-surgically and diagnosis was made on surgical intervention.

Rheumatoid Arthritis

This is a chronic disease characterized by inflammatory changes in the joints and by rarefaction and resorption of bone. The etiology is essentially unknown, but may be auto-immune in nature, even though the disease usually occurs in young people and is much more common in females than it is in males.

Clinical Picture

The early pathology of rheumatoid arthritis may present itself as swelling of the joints with inflammation of the joints and synovial membranes. Inflammation of the capsules of surrounding tissues may be seen in the foot as swollen erythematous areas, red in color and marked by hypertrophy of the villous processes around the joints. In the advanced forms of rheumatoid arthritis, granulation tissue extends over the articular surfaces of the joints with the development of a pannus formation. This pannus formation is usually converted to fibrous tissue which binds the two articular surfaces together to form a fibrous ankylosis of the joint. Rheumatoid nodules are seen in less than 15% of rheumatoids, usually in later stages.

Treatment

Treatment may consist of salicylates, steroids, gold therapy, as well as many other different forms of treatment. The nodular lesions which are seen on the foot seldom need treatment. Surgical excision may be necessary if they are painful. However, the recurrence rate is usually very high.

3. BULLOUS PEMPHIGOID

Bullous pemphigoid may present itself as numerous large, tense bulla and may be chronic or a self-limited condition lasting for a short period of time. These bullous lesions differ from those of pemphigus vulgaris in that the blister-like lesions in bullous pemphigoid do not break as easily and usually these bullae have a tendency to heal after the fluid has been released.

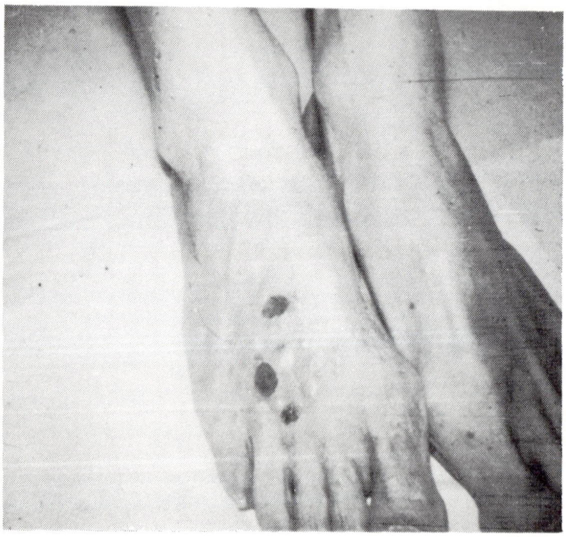

FIGURE 3-22

Bullous Pemphigoid: Uncommon on the foot. May be confused with epidermolysis bullosa. (Courtesy Isidore Zeligman, M.D., Baltimore, Maryland)

Differential Diagnosis

Pemphigus vulgaris, erythema multiforme, dermatitis herpetiformis, epidermolysis bullosa.

Etiology

Bullous pemphigoid is believed to be an auto-immune disease.

Treatment

Treatment usually consists of corticosteroid therapy, although methotrexate has also been utilized in the treatment of bullous pemphigoid.

4. DIABETES MELLITUS

Diabetes is a metabolic disease characterized by an increased amount of blood sugar (hyperglycemia), and an increase in sugar

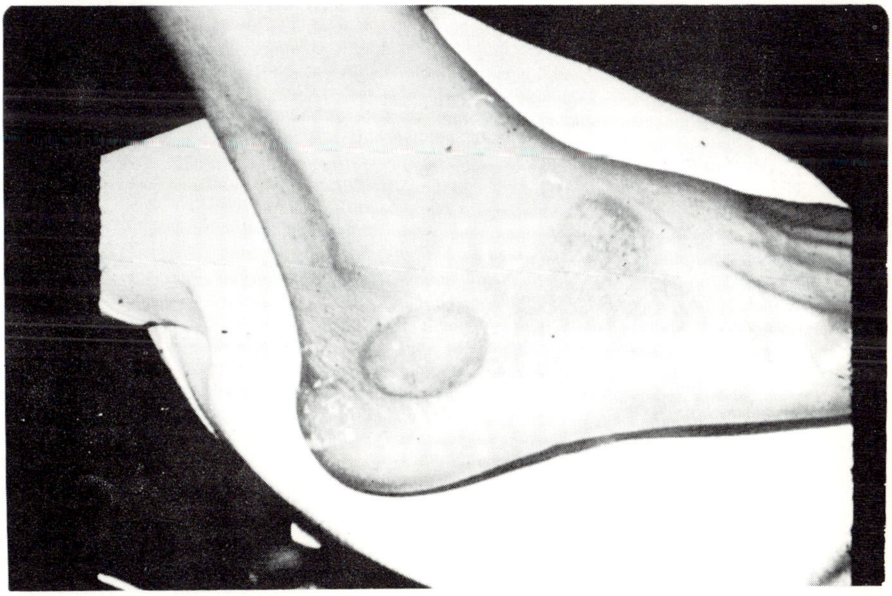

FIGURE 3-23

Fixed Drug Eruption: Not always bullous. Occurs in the same location each time the offending agent is ingested. Succeeding episodes lead to hyperpigmentation of the area. Barbituates and phenophthalein are the most common agents. (Courtesy W. V. R. Shellow, M.D., Los Angeles, California)

in the urine (glycosuria). The cardinal signs of diabetes are generally an elevated blood sugar and the appearance of sugar in the urine. There may be two types of diabetes: the juvenile type and the maturity onset diabetes.

Etiology

Generally, the etiology of diabetes is unknown, however, heredity plays a great role. Signs and symptoms of diabetes are usually pruritis, polyphasia, polyuria and polydipsia.

Treatment

The treatment of diabetes is generally to see that the patient lives a normal life and has a diet for his normal needs. If diet alone cannot be effective in the treatment of diabetes, various forms of hyperglycemic drugs should be utilized in establishing an equal balance of sugar and insulin within the body.

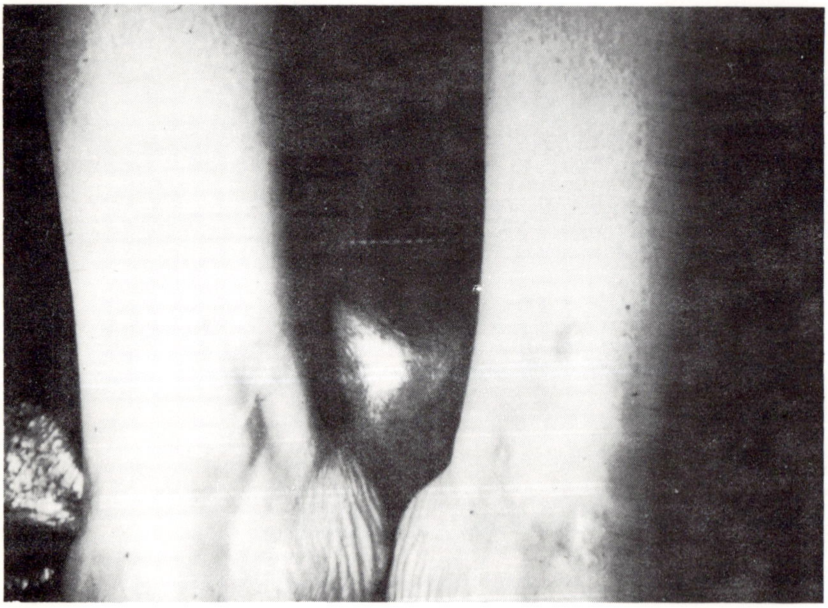

FIGURE 3-24

Necrobiosis Lipoidica Diabeticorum: These lesions are rare manifestation in diabetes mellitus. (Courtesy Isidore Zeligman, M.D., Baltimore, Maryland)

Granuloma annulare

Granuloma annulare is a chronic benign dermatoses of unknown etiology. Characteristically, it is usually seen in children and young adults and may present itself as a ring type of lesion, which may vary from one to several centimeters. The presence of these lesions may suggest the possibility of rheumatoid arthritis as well as diabetes mellitus.

Treatment

These lesions have a tendency to spontaneously disappear. Various forms of treatment, ranging from X-ray therapy to surgical excision have been utilized, however, intralesional injections of corticosteriods have recently proved perhaps to be the best mode of therapy, if treatment is necessary.

Necrobiosis lipoidica diabeticorum

This is a rare manifestation of diabetes, and may only be seen in two percent of diabetic patients. These lesions are usually atrophic, yellowish, depressed areas with telangiectatic blood vessels running through the course of the lesion. Patients of any age may be affected, and the lesions are most frequently seen on the extremities. These lesions are usually asymptomatic and the main problem seems to be that of appearance. It is sometimes ulcerative and this can be very painful.

Treatment

General therapy is usually not successful, however, the intralesional injections of corticosteriods have been helpful.

Xanthoma diabeticorum

This is generally a rare complication of diabetes which may present itself as crops of papules or nodules which may appear almost anywhere on the body and extremities. These papules are usually yellowish in nature, but may show reddened areas surrounding the lesions. These lesions may be tender and may itch. Elevation of the serum triglycerides is present.

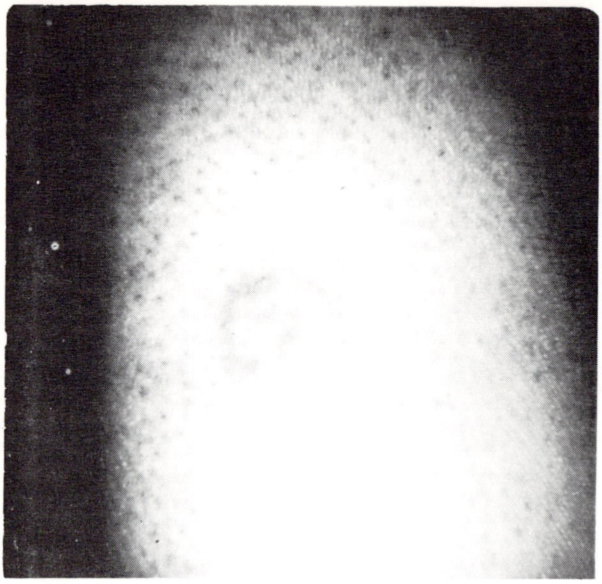

FIGURE 3-25

Xanthoma Diabeticorum: Localized discrete yellowish firm nodular lesion of lower leg.

Treatment

The treatment of these lesions usually rests on the treatment of the underlying diabetes and hyperlipemia and usually the lesions disappear with proper treatment. Other lesions which may present themselves in diabetes may be: malperforan ulcers, diabetic gangerene, diabetic dermopathy.

5. ERYTHEMA ELEVATUM DIUTINUM

Erythema elevatum diutinum may present itself as persistent nodular and plaque-like lesions, usually seen on the extremities. It is very rare on the foot.

Etiology

The etiology of this disease is essentially unknown, however, it may be due to a hypersensitivity reaction.

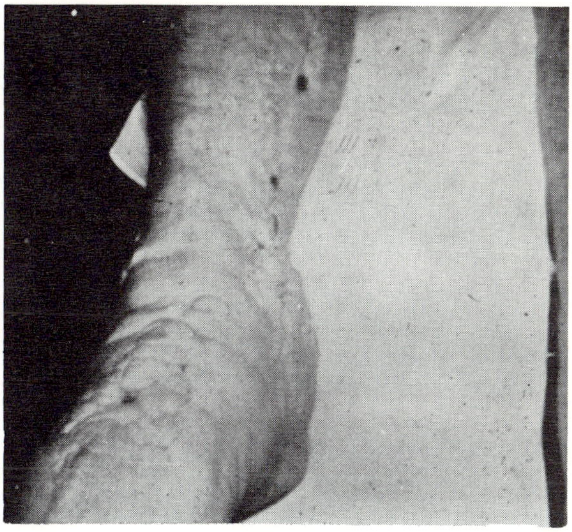

FIGURE 3-26

Xanthoma: Severe lesions of foot and leg due to thyroid disorder. (Courtesy Sanford Rosenfeld, D.P.M., Detroit, Michigan)

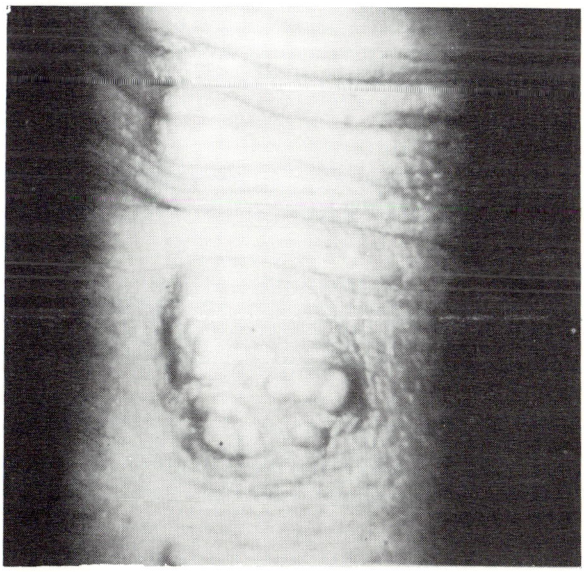

FIGURE 3-27

Xanthoma Diabeticorum — Isolated lesions over achilles tendon.

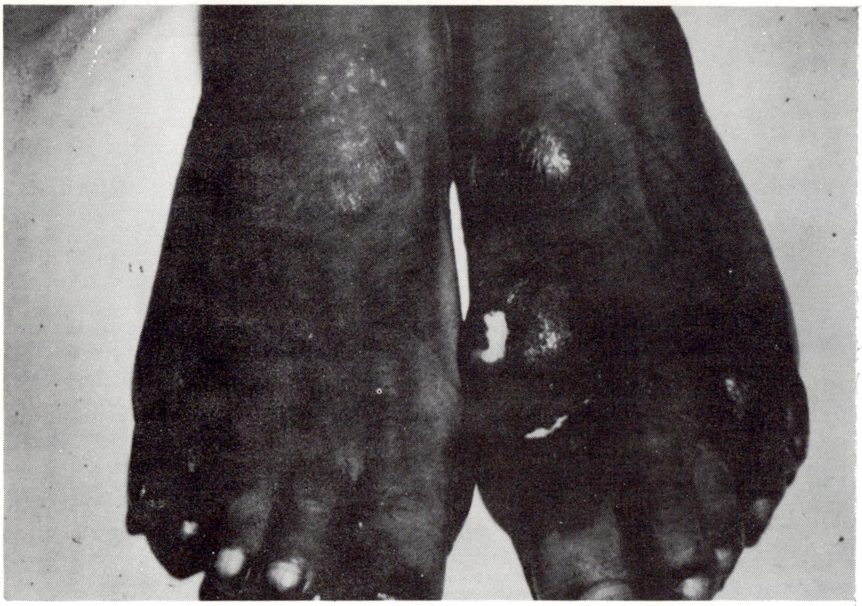

FIGURE 3-28

Erythema Elevatum Diutinum — This is a rare eruption characterized by persistant nodular and plaque like lesions chiefly on the extremities. Microscopically, it has features suggesting a necrotizing vasculitis, and may be a form of hypersensitivity reaction. (Courtesy of W. V. R. Shellow, M.D., Los Angeles, California)

Clinical Picture

These lesions are usually multiple in nature and when they occur on the foot are usually seen on the extensor surfaces. They are usually symmetrically located on the foot and present themselves as nodules and plaques showing various degrees of infiltration and elevation above the skin. The lesions vary in color, ranging from red in the earlier stages of the condition, to dark purple-like lesions in the later stages. Microscopic examination of biopsy reveals vasculitis.

Symptoms

These lesions may present no symptoms other than occasional itching, or they may develop severe pain and tenderness. Gouty arthritis has also been associated with this disease.

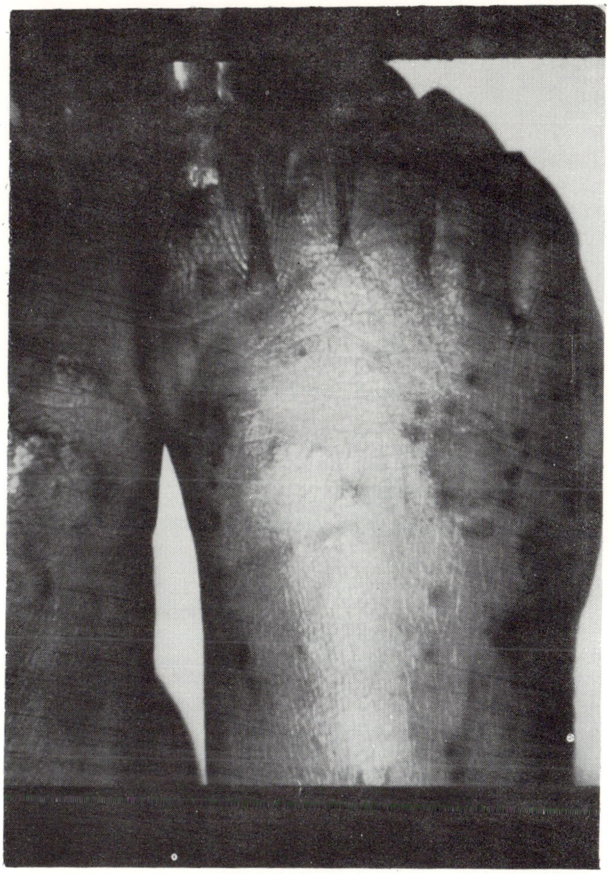

FIGURE 3-29

Vasculitis: May have protean manifestations, including papules, nodules, and ulcers. Differential diagnosis: sarcoidosis, tuberculosis, syphilis, trichinosis. (Courtesy W. V. R. Shellow, M.D., Los Angeles, California)

Treatment

Treatment is usually symptomatic; however, in general, treatment is usually unsatisfactory.

6. MASTOCYTOSIS SYNDROME

Mastocytosis is a term used to describe a condition characterized by an accumulation of mast cells in various organs of the body. When mast cells are limited to the skin, this condition is known as urticaria pigmentosa. However, when the lesions occur as a single infiltration of the dermis, an isolated mastocytoma may be noted. These cutaneous lesions may occur at any age, but they more commonly occur during early infancy and childhood. The childhood form usually involutes spontaneously, but the adult form persists.

Etiology

The etiology of this condition is essentially unknown.

Treatment

The treatment of mastocytoma depends on the stages of the condition, and excision may be utilized for isolated lesions. It is known, however, that these lesions may completely involute spontaneously after a few years without any association of systemic disease.

7. MYCOBACTERIAL INFECTIONS

There are various forms of mycobacterial infections which may present lesions of the foot. The most common types of mycobacterial infections are:

1. mycobacterium tuberculosis
2. mycobacterium bovis
3. mycobacterium leprae
4. mycobacterium marinum

However, in the United States, the most common lesion seen is that of the swimming pool granuloma, which is caused by mycobacterium marinum.

Treatment

Treatment is usually symptomatic and most lesions may heal without therapy. However, systemic and intralesional anti-tuberculosis therapy has been utilized, as have local heat, X-rays, and surgical excision.

8. MYCOSIS FUNGOIDES

(Granuloma fungoides, multiple sarcoma of the skin)

Mycosis fungoides is a malignant proliferation of the reticulo-endothelial cells of the skin with unknown etiology. Some au-

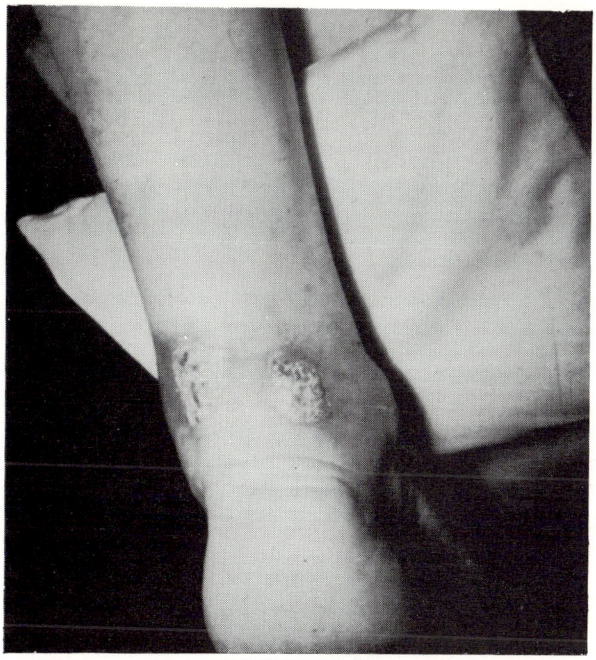

FIGURE 3-30

Mycobacterium Marinum Granuloma: Commonly known as a swimming pool granuloma. (Courtesy Isidore Zeligman, M.D., Baltimore, Maryland)

thors classify it with malignant lymphomas,[21] while others list it under malignant reticuloses.[76] The average duration is about 20 years, and most patients are over 60 years of age when death occurs. In some cases, the disease progresses into an internal reticulo-malignancy such as Hodgkin's disease or leukemia.[76]

This disease was first described in 1806 by Alibert,[1] who, in 1832, names mycosis fungoide because of the mushroom-like appearance of the tumors. In 1959, Bluefarb reviewed 308 cases from the literature; he found 57.5% of the patients were males, the average age of onset was 49.2 years, with the disease being more common in caucasians, and 27% of the patients presented lesions on the lower extremities, while 16% presented a generalized distribution.[6]

Clinical Picture

The clinical picture of mycosis fungoides has many variations. It is generally discussed in three stages, although these stages may vary and one or more may never be present.

The first stage usually consists of an *intensely* pruritic, eczematous, yellow-to-red patch with concave borders. These lesions tend to disappear and recur, and are refractory to the therapy. The patient may have fever and arthralgia. The clinician should be suspicious that any pruritic para-psoriatic patch on the foot may indicate mycosis fungoides because in the more common cause of such patches, the feet are spared.[79]

In the second, or infiltrative stage, the typical lesion is a granular or wart-like patch with a red, tense, shiny surface and surrounded by a purplish ring. These lesions may progress into extensive ulcerations or disappear leaving atrophy and pigmentation. New lesions continue to appear throughout this stage, and generalized lymph-adenopathy may be present.

The third stage is the true tumor stage. Small, subcutaneous nodules occur at the site of a previous infiltrative lesion. These tumors enlarge rapidly and have a marked tendency to ulcerate. When extensive ulceration occurs, a generalized toxemia and cachexia develops and death usually ensues. Rare spontaneous remissions have been reported.

Differential Diagnosis

Differential diagnosis is very difficult and can mimic many skin diseases but varies depending on the stage of the disease. Usually the diagnosis is made histologically when the skin lesions do not respond to treatment.

Treatment

Therapy is palliative rather than curative. Radiation therapy may cause the lesions to regress, but they invariably recur. Topical corticosteroids, nitrogen mustard and similar drugs have been helpful in giving long term remissions. Some specialists believe a cure may lie in the perfection of bone marrow homo-transplants.[79]

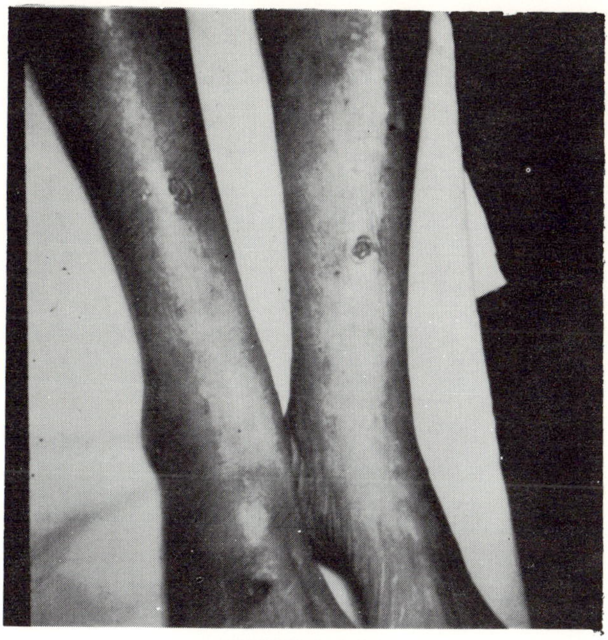

FIGURE 3-31

Lymphoma: Tumor stage of lymphoma should be differentiated from any of the granulomas. Differential diagnosis should include mycosis fungoides and Hodgkins disease. (Courtesy of Isidore Zeligman, M.D., Baltimore, Maryland)

9. PAPULO — SQUAMOUS DISEASES

Psoriasis

Psoriasis is mentioned because it is a common disorder which is believed hereditary in nature. Its etiology is essentially unknown, even though endocrine infections, metabolic and psychogenic factors may have some relationship to this entity. There are several forms of psoriasis, however, the most common, found on the plantar surface of the foot, are those of hyperkeratotic psoriatic lesions; also interdigital psoriasis and pustular psoriasis, which is usually localized to the soles. Psoriatic nail changes and psoriatic arthritis may be seen in the distal joints.

Even though psoriasis is not a definite tumorous condition of the foot, psoriatic lesions often present themselves to the clinician who might misdiagnose psoriasis as a various form of neoplasm. Treatment is often unsatisfactory.

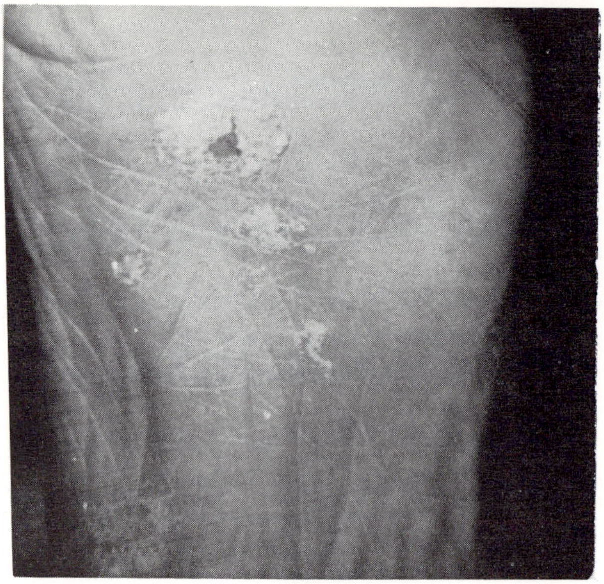

FIGURE 3-32

Psoriasis: Psoriatic lesions on the plantar surface of the foot often take on hyperkeratotic appearance in the formation of plaques. Pustular forms are often frequently seen and frequently confused with tinea pedis.

Lichen Planus

Lichen planus is an inflammatory dermatitis essentially of unknown etiology. The characteristic lesions on the skin may represent themselves as small, flat topped violaceous papules. Other lesions of lichen planus may be atrophic or hypertrophic. Lichen planus lesions on the sole resemble those of callous formation because the lesions have a tendency to coalesce and thicken. The treatment of lichen planus is essentially symptomatic, including topical and intralesional corticosteroids.

10. PARASITIC INFECTIONS

The most common of the parasitic infections affecting the foot is known as cutaneous larva migrans, commonly called the "creeping eruption". This condition is usually seen in the Southeastern.

portions of the United States as well as in Central America, and in tropical areas of the world. There may be various etiologic agents of larva migrans, the most common being Anyclostoma braziliense and A. caninum. "Creeping eruption" may affect any exposed portion of the body.

Clinical Picture

After the invasion of the parasite, inflammation of the area may develop, characterized by chronic pruritis and erythema surrounding the general area. If the infection is allowed to maintain itself for any long period of time, severe skin involvement may develop.

Treatment

Understanding the nature of the condition, and prevention of development of such a condition, are primary concerns. The old-

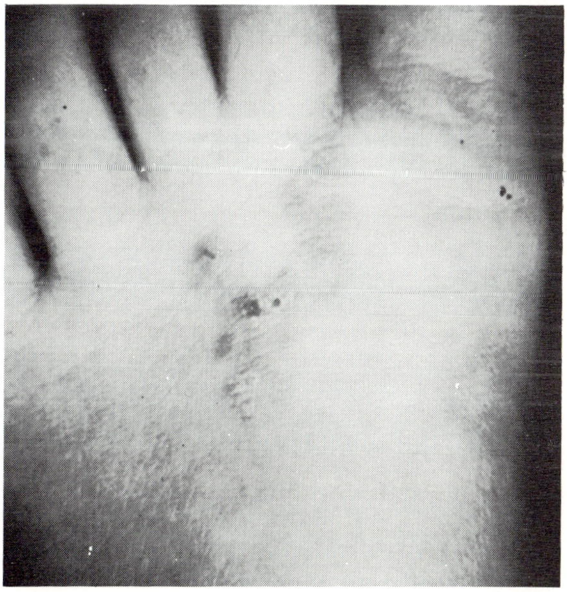

FIGURE 3-33

Creeping Eruption (Cutaneous Larval Migrans) Occurs in the southern United States, commonly in children. Caused by larvae of cat) Ancylostoma braziliense) and dog hookworms (Ancylostoma Cainum), etc.

est method of treatment, however, is that of cryotherapy (liquid nitrogen or the application of dry ice) particularly to the most distal aspects of the cutaneous involvement. Systemic drugs, such as hetrazan and thiabendazole, have been effective in the treatment of "creeping eruption."

11. REITER'S SYNDROME

Reiter's Syndrome is a syndrome which usually occurs in young males, and rarely occurs in females.

Etiology

The etiology of Reiter's Syndrome is essentially unknown.

Clinical Picture

Clinically the symptoms are non-specific urethritis, conjunctivitis, and an asymmetrical arthritis of the major weight bearing joints. The symptoms may present themselves at one time or separately. Reiter's Syndrome has been known to develop, due to bacillary dysentary and sexual contact. Some believe that a virus or mycoplasma may also be the etiological agent. Cutaneous lesions may manifest themselves on the foot, and these lesions are commonly known as keratosis blennorrhagica. Onycholysis may also develop in which there are various degrees of thickening and dystrophy of the nails which may eventually be shed.

Differential Diagnosis

Differential diagnosis includes serum sickness, rheumatoid arthritis, gouty arthritis, gonococcal arthritis, and especially psoriatic arthritis.

Treatment

The treatment of the condition includes anti-inflammatory agents, methotrexate, and antibiotic therapy may be used for the urethritis. Systemic administration of corticosteriods are also utilized in occular involvement and for the arthritis.

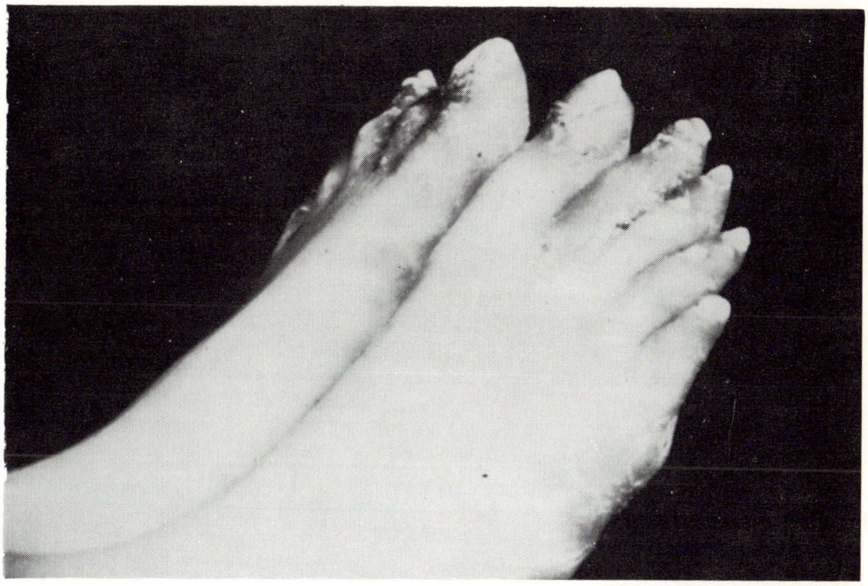

FIGURE 3-34

Keratodermia Blenorrhagica. This is a rare dermatosis seen in Reiter's Syndrome. Lesions may appear as horny pustular crusted lesions. (Courtesy Isidore Zeligman, M.D., Baltimore, Maryland)

12. SYPHILIS

Syphilis is divided into three clinical stages. 1) primary, 2) secondary, and 3) tertiary. The primary lesion of syphilis is that of the chancre which develops at the site of innoculation and the penetration of the skin by the infecting organism. The classical form of chancre is usually single, round, pea or dime size in shape and is painless and is usually elevated above the surrounding tissue. It is usually located on the genitalia, but extragenital chancres are becoming more common. Secondary syphilis usually develops about six weeks after the primary resolves. A generalized eruption may be dark red, indurated, macular-papular, or papular-squamous in nature on the soles. On occasion it may also be pustular. It is in the secondary stage of syphilis that lesions of the palms and soles of the feet are usually seen. Alopecia and generalized lymphadenopathy may also be seen. In the tertiary stage of syphilis, various forms of trophic ulcers of the feet may be present. This is often seen in tabes dorsalis. Cutaneous gummas are another manifestation of late lues. The treatment of this systemic disease is that of anti-syphilitic therapy, as well as symptomatic treatment.

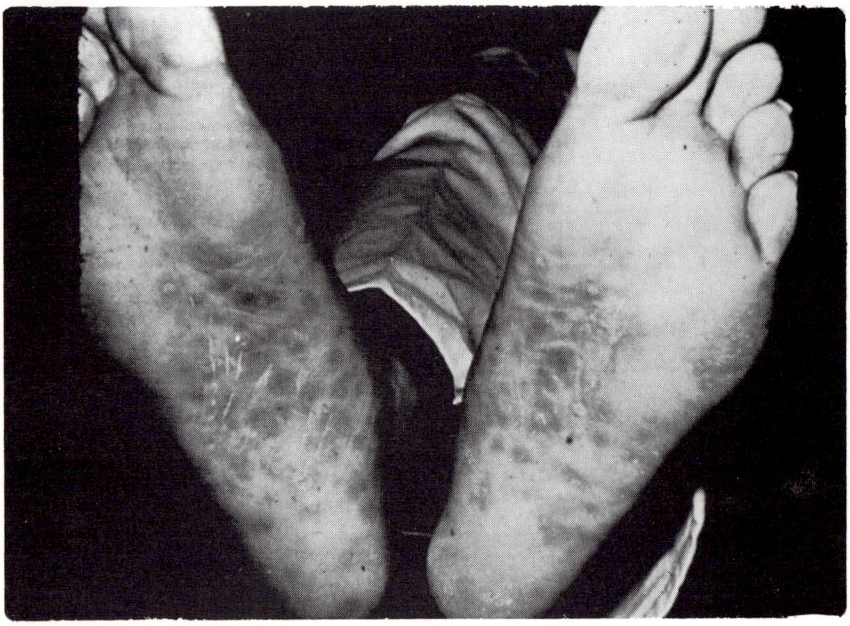

FIGURE 3-35

Secondary syphilis — characteristic papular eruption on the soles. The palms would be diagnostic. (Courtesy W. V. R. Shellow, M.D., Los Angeles, California)

BIBLIOGRAPHY

1. Alibert, J. L. M.: Description des maladies de la peau. Observ. es a l'hospital St. Louis, Paris, Barrois, 1806.
2. Balkin, S. W.: Plantar keratosis: Treatment by injectable liquid silicone — Report on an eight year experience. *Clin. Orthop.*,**87**:235-47, 1972.
3. Balkin, S. W.: Silicone injection for plantar keratosis. *JAPA*,**56**:1966.
4. Baumal, A., et al: Nail bed involvement in phemphigus vulgaris. *Arch Derm;* **107**:751, 1973.
5. Berlin, S. J.: Tropical steroids in intractable plantar keratosis. *JAPA*, **57**:5-8, 1967.

6. Bluefarb, S. M.: *Cutaneous Manifestations of the Malignant Lymphomas.* Thomas, Springfield, Ill., 1959.
7. Bonovilla, E. F.: Histopathology of the heloma durum: some significant features and their implications. *JAPA,* **58**:423, 1965.
8. Bronston, G.: A soft tissue approach for plantar lesions. *JAPA,* **57**:331, 1967.
9. Brown, F. C.: Punctate keratoderma. *Arch. Dermatol.,* **104**:682-3, 1971.
10. Brunsting, L., Kierland, R., Perry, H., Winkelmann, R., and Muller, S.: Palmar plantar hyperkeratosis with periodontosis (Papillon - Lefevre syndrome), presented before Minnesota Dermatologic Society, 1963. *Arch. Derm.,* (Chicago) **90**:330, 1964.
11. Buchanan, R. N., Jr.: Keratosis punctata palmaris et plantaris. *Arch. Derm.,* (Chicago) **88**:644-50, 1963.
12. Butterworth, T. and Strean, L. P.: *Clinical Genodermatology.* Williams and Wilkins Pub. Co., 1962.
13. Callan, N. J.: Circumscribed palmoplantar keratoderma. *Australias J. Dermatol* **11**:76-81, 1970.
14. Cannon, A. B.: Arsenical Dermatitis followed by keratosis and alopecia. *Arch. Dermat. and Syph.,* **24**:676, 1931.
15. Carrel, J. M.: Pemphigus vulgaris: Report of a case and a review of the differential diagnosis. *JAMA* **62**:183-6, 1972.
16. Chalmers, A. J. and Kamar, A.: Keratodermia punctata. *J. Trop. Med.,* **20**:121, 1917.
17. Chung, H.: Keratosis palmaris et plantaris hereditarian. *Arch. Dermat. and Syph.,* **36**:303-313, 1937.
18. Clendenning, W. E., et al: Mycosis Fungoides. *Arch. Derm.,* **89**:785, 1964.
19. Cockayne, E. A.: Inherited abnormalities of the skin and its appendages. *London, Oxford University Press,* 1933.
20. Conklin, D. E.: Hyperkeratosis. *JAMA,* **169**:1694, 1959.
21. Conway, H., Hugo, N., and Tulenko, J.: *Surgery of Tumors of the Skin* Charles C. Thomas Publishers, Springfield, Illinois, 1966.
22. Curth, H. O.: In discussion on Garb, J.: Diagnosis, acanthosis Nigricans (juvenile type). Presented before Bronx Dermatological Society, 1959, *Arch. Derm.* **81**:1005, 1960.
23. Darier, R. J. and co-workers: *Nouvelle Pratique Dermatologique,* Vol. 6, Masson, Paris, 1936.
24. Davies-Colley, N.: Disseminated clavus of the hands and feet. *Trans. Path. Soc. London,* **30**:451, 1879.
25. Davis, C. M.: Keratosis palmaris et Plantaris. Presented before Philadelphia Derm. Society, *J. Cut. Dis.,* **27**:168, 1909.
26. Dickson, M.: Keratosis palmaris et plantaris: A case report. *JAPA,* **56**:376, 1966.
27. Eller, J. J.: *Tumors of the Skin,* Lea and Febiger, October, 1939.
28. Everall, J.: Tylosis palmaris et paltaris with unusual bullous lesions. *Brit. J. Derm.,* **66**:54, 1954.
28A. Fitzpatrick, et al: *Dermatology in General Medicine.* McGraw-Hill Inc.
29. Fox, G. H.: Congenital diffuse Keratosis. Presented before N.Y. Derm. Society, *J. Cut. Dis.,* **29**:22, 1911.
30. Fred, H. L., et al: Keratosis palmaris et plantaris. *Arch. Intern. Med.* (Chicago), **113**:866-71, 1964.
31. Galanter, D. R.: Hyperkeratosis palmoplantaris and periodontosis; the Papillon — LeFevre Syndrome. *J. Periodont.,* **40**:40-7, 1969.

32. Costello, M. and Gibbs, R. C.: *The Palms and Soles in Medicine.,* Charles C. Thomas Publishers, Springfield, Illinois, 1967, pp. 523-525.
33. Gomez, O. J., et al: Palmo-plantar hyperkeratosis, diffuse and circumscribed. (Thost-unna type). *Int. J. Dermatol,* **11**:96-105, April-June, 1972.
34. Gorlin, R. J., et al: The syndrome of palmar-plantar hyperkeratosis and premature periodontal destruction of the teeth. *J. Pediat.,* **65**:895-908, December, 1964.
35. Graham, F. H., et al: Chemistry of Bowen's Disease: Relationship to arsenic, *J. Invest. Derm.,* **37**:317, 1961.
36. Gray, A. M. H.: A case of cornua cutanea of the feet. *Proc. Roy. Soc. Med.* **13**:57, 1920.
37. Greither, A.: Keratosis palmo-plantaris with periodontopathies (Papillon - LeFevre). *Dermatologica.,* **119**:248-263, 1959.
38. Gunther, S. H.: Vitamin A acid in treatment of palmoplantar kerotoderma: Clinical investigations and experience results with 13 patients. *Arch. Dermatol.,* **106**:854-7, 1972.
39. Hadida, E., et al: Palmoplantar keratoderma: Role of chronic occupational contact with arsenic. *Bull. Soc. Fr. Syphiligr.,* **79**:287-8, 1972 (F).
40. Hagashima, M., et al: Keratosis palmo-plantaris diffusa: A type with so-called granular degeneration. *Keio. J. Med.,* **19**:205-11, 1970.
41. Hall, A. F.: Arsenical keratoses disappearing with vitamin A therapy. Presented before Los Angeles dermatological society, 1944. *Arch. Dermat. and Syph.* **53**:154, 1946.
42. Headington, J. T.: Mixed tumors of skin-eccrine and apocrine types. *Arch. Derm.,* **84**:989, 1961.
43. Heiss, H. B., et al: Keratosis palmaris et plantaris treatment with topically applied Vitamin A, Acid. *Arch. Derm.,* (Chicago), **101**:100-3, 1970.
44. Hertforth, A., et al: Juvenile periodontopathies and skin diseases. *Dtsch. Zahnaerzti. Z.,* **20**:242-6, 1973.
45. Hermel, M. B., et al: Keratoderma palmaris et plantaris: Roentgenologic aspects. *Radiology,* **92**:1101-2, 1969.
46. Holevich, Y.: Surgical treatment of palmar and plantar keratosis. *Acta. Chir. Plast.,* (Praha) **9**:34-42, 1967.
47. Hovorka, O., and Ehlers, E.: Mal de Meleda, *Arch. of Dermat. and Syph.* **40**:1897, Abstracted *Brit. J. Derm.,* **9**416, 1897.
48. Isaacs, B.: Keratodermia palmaris et plantaris. *Glasgow Med. J.,* **31**:175, 1950.
49. Jacobson, J. P. and Anderson, N. P.: Callosities, multiple congenital. Presented before Los Angeles Derm. Society, 1942. *Arch. Dermat. and Syph.* **47**:288, 1943.
50. Keir, M.: Keratoderm plantaris et palmaris. *Brit. J. Derm.,* **79**:419-21, 1967.
51. Kierland, R. R.: Acanthosis nigricans: An analysis of data in twenty-two cases and a study of it frequency in necropsy material. *J. Invest. Derm.,* **9**:299, 1947.
52. Kisher, W. H.: Keratosis palmaris et plantaris. *Plast. Reconstr. Surg.,* **51**:424-7, 1973.
53. Klaus, S., et al: Localized epidermolytic hyperkeratosis. A form of keratoderma of the palms and soles. *Arch. Derm.* (Chicago), **101**:272-5, 1970.
54. Lapidus, P. W.: Orthopedic skin lesions of the soles and the toes. Cal-

louses, corns, plantar warts, keratomas, neurovascular growths, onychomas. *Clin. Ortho.,* **45**:87-100, 1967.
55. Levy, H.: Multiple keratoncanthoma. Presented before N.Y. Academy of Medicine, 1964. *Arch. Derm.* (Chicago), **83**:1030, 1961.
56. Lieberthal, D.: In discussion on Zeisler, E. P.: Congenital keratosis of palms and soles. *J. Cut. Disease,***37**:262, 1919.
57. Mackee, George and Cipollano, Anthony: *Cutaneous Cancer and Precancer.*Lancaster Press Inc. Pa., 1937.
58. Masson, J. C. and Montgomery, H.: Acanthosis nigricans and pelvis malignancy, *Proc. Staff Meeting,* Mayo Clinic, **11**:113-117, 1936.
59. Michael, J. C.: Keratoderma disseminatum palmaris et plantaris. *Arch. Derm. and Syph.,* **27**:78-88, 1933.
60. Miller, J. Q., et al: A specific congenital brain defect (Arinencephaly) in 13-15 trisomy. *New Eng. J. Med.,* **268**:120, 1963.
61. Miller, W. A.: Fasciotomy in the treatment of plantar keratosis and other conditions of the foot. *J. Okla. State Med. Assoc.,* **66**:13-7, 1973.
62. Montgomery, R. M., and Montgomery, A. H.: Common hyperkeratotic lesions of the foot. *JAMA,* **124**:756, 1944.
63. Montgomery, R. M.: Painful Cutaneous lesions of the feet. *Southern Med., J.,* **63**:615-9, 1970.
64. Neubauer, O.: Arsenical cancer; A review. *British Journal of Cancer,* **1**:192, 1947.
65. Nexmand, P. H.: Keratoderma palmare et plantare disseminatum with special reference to its mode of inheritance and the influence of mechanical factors on its development. *Dermatologic,* **99**(2):157, 1949.
66. Niles, H. D., and Klumpp, M. M.: Mal de Meleda. *Arch. Dermat. and Syph.* **39**:409-421, 1939.
67. Ollondorff, C. H.: Cancer associated with acanthosis nigricans. *Arch. Surg.* **47**:517-552, 1943
68. Olmstead, H. C.: Keratodermia plantaris et palmaris congenitalis. *Amer. J. Dis. Child.* **133**:757, 1927.
69. Onderstall, W. J.: Hyperkeratosis of soles. *Proc. Mine. Med. Off. Assoc.* **50**:41-2, 1970.
70. Parounagian, M.: Keratosis palmaris et plantaris hereditarium. Presented before Manhattan Derm. Society, 1913. *J. Cut. Dis.,* **32**:462, 1914.
71. Penred, V.: Hereditary keratosis or tylosis palmae. *Brit. Med. J.* **1**:1132, 1898.
72. Perrot, H., et al: Palmoplantar keratosis of Dariers Disease and multiple abnormalities. (Ultrastructural study). *Ann. Dermatol. Syphiligr.* (Paris) **98**:153-60, 1971.
73. Pollitzer, S.: Internat. Atlas self-hautkr. 10 (1890)
74. Pollitzer, S.: Acanthosis Nigricans. *JAMA,* **53**:1369-1373, 1909.
75. Raphael, A., et al: Hyperkeratosis of gingival and plantar surfaces. *Periodontics,* **6**:118-20, June, 1968.
76. Reed, R. J. and Cummings, C. E.: Malignant reticuloses and related conditions of the skin. *Cancer,* **19**:1231, 1966.
77. Robbin, Gerald M.: Atypical Callous — A Case Report. *JAPA,* **60**:212-213, 1970.
78. Robbins, Stanley L.: *Pathology,*W. B. Saunders Co., 1967.
79. Rook, A., Wilkenson, D. S., and Eibling, A. J. G.: *Textbook of Dermatology,* Davis, Phila., 1968.
80. Rook, A. and Moffatt, J. L.: Multiple self-healing epithelioma of Ferguson Smith types. *Arch. Derm.,* (Chicago), **74**:525, 1956.

81. Ross, J. B.: Keratosis punctata. *Brit. J. Derm.,* **75**:478-83, 1963.
82. Rosset, M.: Arsenical keratosis associated with carcinomas of the internal organs. Case report. *Canadian Med. Assoc. J.,b6 78*:416, 1958.
83. Rothman, S.: Letters to the editor, differences in types of keratinization anomalies. *Arch. Derm.,* **87**:2, 1963.
84. Rothman, S.: In discussion on Lorincz, A. L.; Keratoma hereditarium dissipatum palmare et plantare with cutaneous horn formation (Brauer) treated with lithium bromide. *Arch. Derm. and Syph.,* **68**:91 1953.
85. Ruiz-Maldonado, R.: Palmo-plantar hyperkeratosis with periodontosis (Papillon-LeFevre syndrome). *Int. J. Dermatol.,* **10**:10-2, 1961.
86. Samitz, M. H., and Dana, A. S.: *Cutaneous Lesions of the Lower Extremities.* J. B. Lippincott Co., Phila., Pa., 1971.
87. Schaffer, A. W., et al: Hyperkeratosis palmoplantaris with periodontosis (Papillon-Lefevre syndrome) report of a case. *Oral Surg.,* **24**:180-5, 1967.
88. Schwartz, L., Tulipar, L., and Birmingham, D.: *Occupational Diseases of the Skin,* 3rd ed. Lea and Febiger, Phila., 1957, page 84.
89. Scott, M. J., Costello, M. J., and Simuangoo, S.: Keratosis punctata palmaris et plantaris. *Arch. Derm. and Syph.,* **64**:301-308, 1951.
90. Shaw, W. M., Mason, E. H., and Katz, F. G.: Hypothroidism, liver damage and vitamin A deficiency as factors in hyperkeratosis. *Arch. ofDerm. and Syph.,* **66**:197, 1952.
91. Siemens, H. W.: Keratosis palmo-plantaris striata. *Arch. Derm. and Syph.* **157**:392, 1929.
92. Silberberg, F., Kopf, A., and Baer, R. L.: Recurrent keratoacanthoma of the lip. *Arch. Derm.,* **86**:92, 1962.
93. Sommers, S. C., and McManus, R. C.: Multiple arsenical cancers of the skin and internal organs. *Cancer,* **6**:347, 1953.
94. Sommerville, J. and Milne, J. A.: Familiar primary self-healing squamous epitheliumn of the skin. *Brit. J. Dermat. and Syph.,* **62**:483, 1950.
95. Spray, J. B.: Tumors of the lower extremity. *J. Am. Pod. Assoc.,* **62**:207-11, 1972.
96. Stout, A. P. and Cooley, S. C.: Carcinoma of sweat glands. *Cancer,* **4**:521, 1951.
97. Sulzberger and Wolf: *Dermatology.* Year Book Inc., Chicago, 1952.
98. Sutton, Richard L.: *Diseases of the Skin,* C. V. Mosby, Co., 1935.
99. Taub, J. and Steinberg, M.: Porokeratosis plantaris discreta, a previously unrecognized dermatopathological entity. *Int. J. Derm.,* **9**:83-90, 1970.
100. Thomsen, K.: Pustulosis palmaris et plantaris treated with methotrexate. *Acta. Derm. Venereol.* (Stockh.), **51**:397-400, 1971.
101. Tulipan, L.: Keratosis palmaris et plantaris. Presented before the N.Y. Academy of Med. section of Derm. and Syph., 1931, *Arch. Dermat. and Syph.* **24**:140, 1931.
102. Weidman, F.: In discussion on Cross, T., and Schamberg, J.: Symmetrical keratoderma of the extremities (prob. acquired). Presented before Phila. Derm. Soc., 1929. *Arch. Dermat. and Syph.,* **20**:249, 1929.
103. Weisfeld, M. J.: Understanding porokeratosis plantaris discreta. *Am. Pod. Assoc.,* **63**:138-44, 1973.
104. Wiener, Kurt: *Skin Manifestations of Internal Disorders.* C. V. Mosby, Co., St. Louis, 1947.
105. Wise, F.: Paraffin Keratosis and epithelioma, presented before Manhattan Derm. Society, 1930. *Arch. Dermat. and Syph.* **22**:546, 1930.
106. Zaias, N., et al: Pitted keratolysis. *Arch. Derm.* (Chicago), **92**:152-4, 1965.

SECTION IV

NEVI AND MALIGNANT SKIN LESIONS OF THE FOOT

Nevi

INTRODUCTION

Nevus cells are atypical melanocytes derived from normal melanocytes at the epidermal-dermal junction. Melanocytes develop from neural crest tissue in the embryo. They mature and become localized in the skin, eye and pia arachnoid.

At birth, if the melanocytes are present in great number, they can be detected in the dermal portion of the scalp, sacrum and dorsal areas of the hands and feet. They will appear as blue or blue-gray mongolian spots, usually in the sacral area. Mongolian spots are rare in the white race, but are seen in the black and yellow races. Dermal melanocytes that proliferate usually give a circumscribed blue to black lesion called a blue nevus.

The tissue environment of the dermis is unfavorable for the melanocytes so they disappear shortly after birth, but stay at the dermal-epidermal junction for life.[138] At birth, 97% of whites have no nevi. About age two, however, the melanocytes begin to proliferate, usually as tiny brown spots, the first stage in the development of the nevus. They are located at the dermalepidermal junction and are called junctional nevi or said to be at the junctional stage of development.

The nevus has a life cycle with periods of active growth, maturity with quiescence and decline with involution. This cycle generally lasts 50-60 years.[138]

Many people with malignant melanoma have a history of a pre-existing pigmented mole.[88] The pigmented nevus or mole is the most ubiquitous skin tumor in humans with the average adult having about forty.[138] It is readily apparent that the overwhelming percentage of nevi do not develop into melanoma.

This early junctional nevus spreads for a time and as there becomes an increase in the volume of cells, it elevates above the skin. Those on the palms and soles rarely elevate, probably due to the increased thickness of the epidermis in these areas.

As the nevus cells extend into the dermis, the nevus enters the maturity stage and is called a compound nevus. Nevus cells are seen in the dermis and epidermis. During this stage, usually in

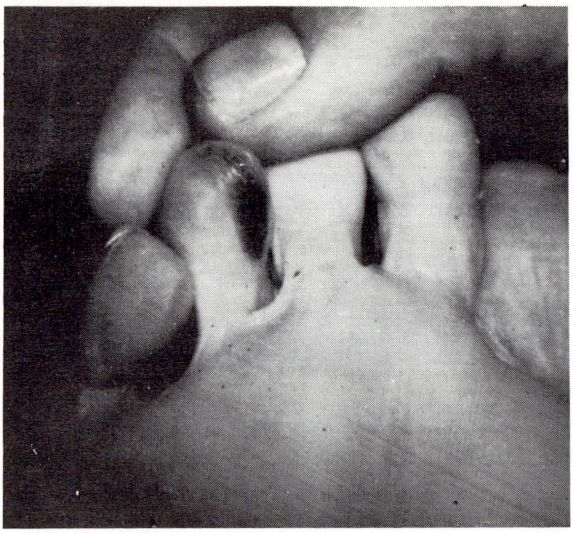

FIGURE 4-1

Large junctional nevi involving 4th toe.

the second decade, the junctional activity or proliferation stops. The melanocytes are no longer producing nevus cells.

In older nevi, the nevus cells are usually confined to the dermis. They are separarted from the epidermis by a band of connective tissue. This is the decline stage for the nevus which is now called an intradermal nevus. This is the least active type of nevus.

The number and size of nevi reach their peak at 20-25 years of age at which time they begin to flatten and fade until they disappear about age 90.[138] This overall life cycle should be kept in mind, and anything not fitting into the picture should be suspect.

Types

Nevi and pigmented lesions of skin are classified by the type of pigmented cell and the position of these cells in the skin.[139] There are six main types of nevi, each with a different clinical significance.

1. *Intradermal nevus*

This is the common mole, and is the most frequently encountered mole in the adult. It is only of cosmetic importance.[100] About 75% of all nevi are the intradermal type. It is uncommon prior to puberty. Clinically, it is a raised, fleshy skin tumor of a tan or light brown color and often contains hair. The intradermal nevus is rarely found on the palms, soles, or genitalia. Histologically, the nevus cells are located in the dermis, and there is no evidence of cellular activity at the junctional zone between the dermis and epidermis. The intradermal nevus has no potential for malignant change.[123]

2. Junctional nevus

The cells lie in the dermal-epidermal junction and show a loss of cohesion and prickling. There is an increased amount of melanin in these cells. In appearance, the junctional nevus is usually hairless, smooth, flat or only slightly raised, and is brown-black to slate in color. It can range in size from two millimeters to several centimeters. It is frequently encountered on the palms, soles and genitalia. According to Potter, the lesion is of significance because about 80% of all melanomas arise from this nevus.[123] Clinically, one would see areas of activity where changes are focal and appear towards the periphery of the lesion. Thus you might find long areas of normal epidermis between areas of involved epidermis.[100]

3. Compound nevus

The cells are located both junctionally and intradermally. Clinically, the lesion is indistinguishable from the intradermal nevus. It is found most commonly in the young adult. About four percent of melanomas arise from compound nevi by virtue of their junctional components.[123]

4. Blue nevus

This occurs most often on the dorsum of the hands and feet and over the face. It is smooth, hairless, and ranges in color from brown to blue-black. Histologically, it is located deep in the dermis and consists of spindle-type cells and fascicles that resemble smooth muscle. The blue nevus seems to manifest a neural origin. A deeply pigmented blue nevus may resemble a melanoma, but a careful history will show that the lesion has been present and remained unchanged for many years. It is uncommon for the blue nevus to become malignant.[123]

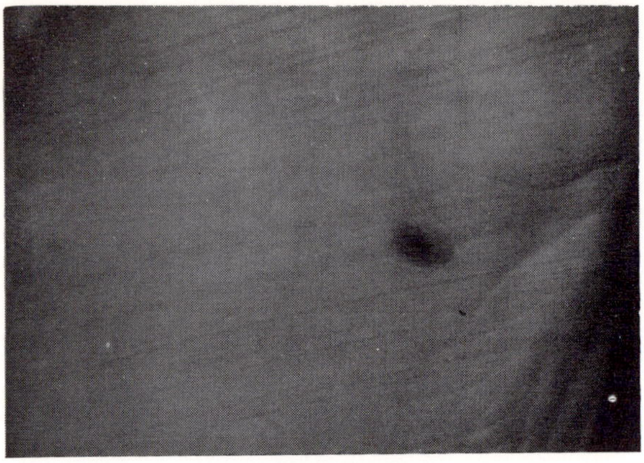

FIGURE 4-2

Compound nevus - plantar surface of foot.

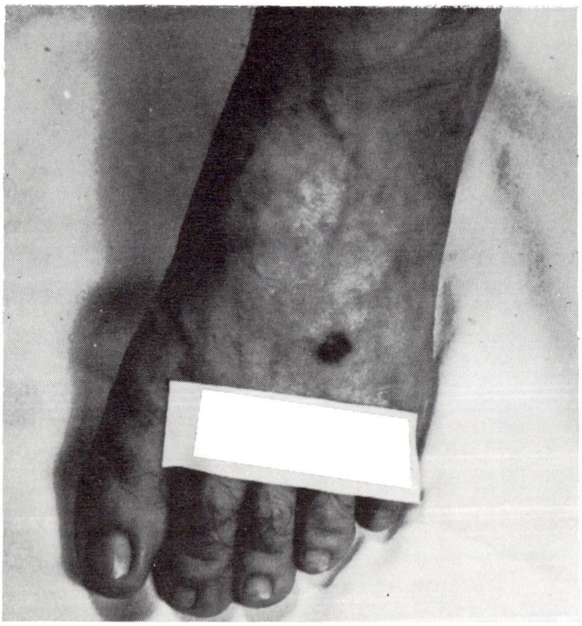

FIGURE 4-3

Blue Nevus dorsum of foot. (Courtesy James Ganley, D.P.M., Norristown, Pa.)

5. Juvenile melanoma

This is unfortunately a poorly named lesion as it is a benign process which occurs predominately in children, but is occasionally found in adults. Its histology mimics the appearance of the true melanoma. In childhood, these lesions almost invariably run a benign course and conservation is indicated in their management. Most lesions in children, which clinically and microscopically appear to be malignant melanomas, are actually these nevi. The microscopic differentiation between the juvenile melanoma and a malignant melanoma in a child requires experience in the pathologic differentiation of these lesions.[123]

6. Mongolian spots

These are seen most frequently in the dark races. They are congenital and are usually found in the sacral area. Clinically, they are circumscribed pigmentations, non-elevated, non-indurated, and dark blue to gray in color. They often disappear spontaneously by the fourth year of life. Microscopically, there are melanocytes deep in the dermis, with the overlying dermis and epidermis being normal. The blue-gray color of the lesion is due to the depth of the brown melanin pigment seen through the overlying skin. They are not pathological and do not undergo malignant change.

TABLE I
THE LIFE OF THE NEVUS[138]

4th Fetal month on	Beginning of some nevi
Birth (Yrs.)	Appearance of first junctional nevi
2	
10	
Puberty	Prepuberty. Appearance of first compound nevi Enlargement and darkening of compound nevi (hormonal stimulation) Appearance of first dermal nevus
20	
Pregnancy	Enlargement and darkening of nevi during pregnancy (Hormonal stimulation)
30	Average number of nevi: 40
	Anytime: Enlargement and darkening of nevi after exogenous ACTH stimulation
40	Gradual loss of pigment
50	
60	Gradual decline in number of nevi
70	
80	Absence of nevi
90	

Melanoma

INTRODUCTION

Malignant melanoma is the malignant lesion of the melanin-producing cell. In the past, it was called a melanosarcoma because it was thought to come from connective tissue elements. At present, it is referred to as a melanocarcinoma or malignant melanoma because pathologists generally agree that it is of ectodermal origin.

There is much discrepancy between the clinical behavior and the histological picture of this highly unpredictable tumor. The differences in the behavior of this tumor often depend on age groups (prepuberty, adult, and elderly), which suggest the rate of endocrine factors, possibly the melanocyte stimulating hormone. In the young, melanoma often runs a very malignant course, while in the elderly, it tends to be fairly benign. Malignant melanomas are rare before 20 years of age.

Three types of melanoma have been distinguished clinically and histologically.[29,87] The lentigo malignant melanoma tends to be the least malignant type. Early in its course it is considered pre-malignant and begins as a small freckle-like lesion. It commonly begins in middle-age and can take as long as thirty years to evolve into an invasive malignancy. Lentigo maligna are found almost exclusively in exposed areas where solar damage is considered the primary etiologic factor. Grossly, it appears as a tan to black flat lesion with some raised portions seen mainly on the face and neck in elderly people. Hutchinson first described this lesion, and it is often referred to as Hutchinson's melanotic freckle.[70] It is very rare in the lower extremities. The superficial spreading melanoma is found anywhere on the body, but is most common on the leg below the knee (especially in females), on the plantar surface of the foot, and on the neck.[86] It is the dominant type in young adults with a high tendency to metastasize and a high mortality rate. Grossly, it is elevated with striking color variations including shades of rose or pink, grey-blue and white with tan or brown as a border.[28] The peak age of occurrence is 56. The most invasive form is the nodular melanoma. This type is metastatic almost from its beginning. It is not associated with exposed areas and is usually seen on the trunk and feet. The prognosis for this type is very grave.

History

Malignant melanoma is a relatively uncommon neoplasm and, at the same time, one of the most unpredictable clinically. About thirty percent of the cases involve the legs and feet. The diagnosis depends ultimately upon the pathologist, but the selection of which nevi to remove and the index of suspicion depends upon the clinician. Too many doctors make a benign diagnosis too readily and close their minds to the possibility of malignant melanoma. We must be constantly aware of this tumor and not waste any time in performing a biopsy on any suspicious nevus.

Hippocrates, in the 5th century B.C., was the first one to record observations on melanoma. Highmore (1651), Bantholin (1677),

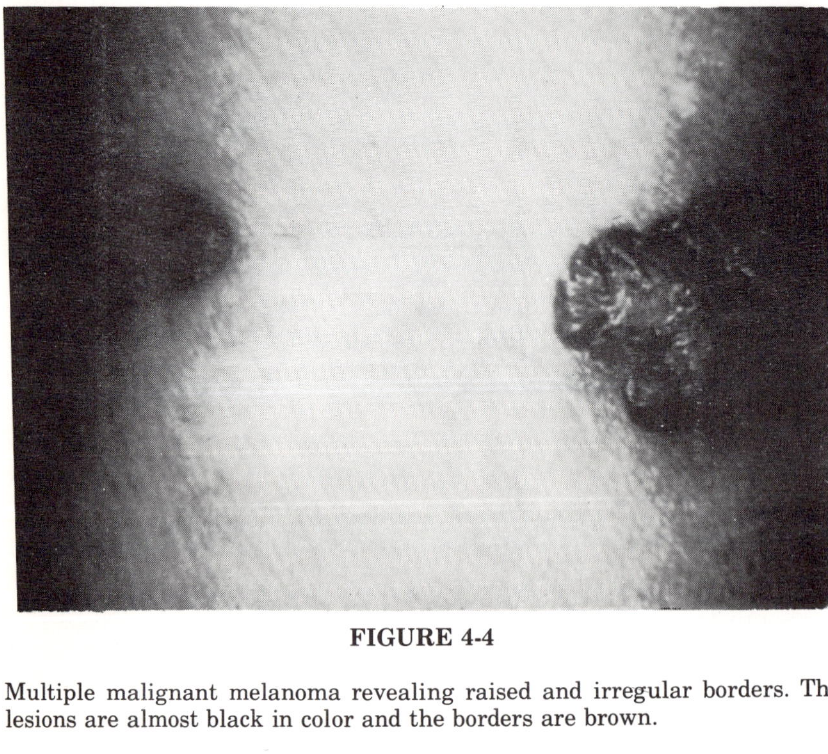

FIGURE 4-4

Multiple malignant melanoma revealing raised and irregular borders. The lesions are almost black in color and the borders are brown.

and Benet (1679) added further descriptions and reports about the lesion they called the "fatal black tumor."[79]

In 1806 Laennec and Dupuytren published separate "Treatise on Melanoma." Carsell (1836) coined the phrase "melanoma" and Pemberton (1858) postulated the spread of melanoma through the lymphatic system and suggested the necessity for lymph node dissection.[79]

The first report of malignant melanoma of the foot was by Langdon in 1894,[82] and articles by Caribet, Moresten, and Hertzler followed at the turn of the century.[131]

In 1907, Herndley described the pathology and recommended wide excision of the primary tumor with lymphadenectomy.[63] In 1908, Pringle expanded the treatment to include excision of skin, subcutaneous tissue, fascia, and areas of spread between the primary tumor and regional lymph nodess.[124]

Klopp (1950) was the first to suggest the use of intra-arterial chemicals in the treatment.[78] Creech (1958) was the first to use perfusion chemotherapy for melanoma of the extremities.[36]

Pack and Gerber (1952) published the most extensive case study to date.[67] Allen and Spitz (1953) published an article in an attempt to correlate clinical and histological variables with prognosis.[2]

Although there has been much written on melanoma throughout history, the basic treatment has not changed drastically in 100 years. Techniques have been reformed and awareness increased, which has lead to improved results over the past 20 years.

Etiology

The actual etiologic factor or factors that will cause a benign nevus to undergo malignant degeneration is unknown. However, there are many predisposing factors referred to in the literature. It is generally accepted that malignant melanomas may come from junctional nevi or junctional components of compound nevi.

The question of trauma as an inciting cause is controversial. Lea, in 1965, compiled 193 cases of malignant melanoma of which 38% gave a history of trauma. He also looked at 530 cases of basal-cell carcinoma of which only 12% gave any history of trauma. He concluded: "The relationship of trauma to the production of malignant melanoma of the skin is regarded as established beyond reasonable doubt."[83] On the other hand, Ghadially, in 1966, experimentally tried to induce malignant changes in nevi found on hamsters and then on fish with similar melanin production to humans, and found that in no case did trauma induce malignant changes. In the case of the hamsters, many of the nevi regressed with trauma.[52]

Excess ultraviolet light or sunlight is an important predisposing factor especially in fair skinned people with blue or green eyes and blonde or red hair. This has been postulated as a genetic predisposition. Also, there are families in which there is a greater incidence of melanoma.[130]

The most likely cause is chronic irritation, ie: on the palms and soles, the digits, and especially around the nails, from shoes, clothing, eye glasses, razors, and belts.[61,88] Nevi in these areas should be closely watched for change.

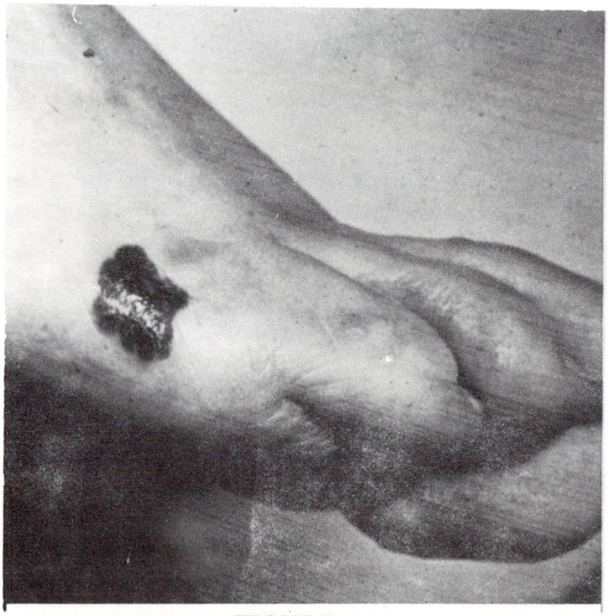

FIGURE 4-5

Malignant melanoma revealing irregular borders on dorsal lateral surface of foot. Approximately 25% of all patients with malignant melanoma relate that a pre-existing pigmented lesion was present. (Courtesy of William V. R. Shellow, M.D., Los Angeles, Calif.)

There is a strong endocrine relationship as evidenced by an increase in the number of cases in pregnant women and in people during the development of secondary sex characteristics.[31] During pregnancy, malignant melanoma metastasize widely and rapidly, having a very poor prognosis.

Jackson, in 1966, reported 25% of all malignant melanoma arise from lentigo maligna (Hutchinson's Freckle), which is a brown-black freckle seen chiefly on the face of the elderly.[73]

There have been rare cases of malignant melanoma forming in vaccination scars, tattoos, in an indelible pencil puncture wound,[77] and, in one case, from a long-standing intradermal nevus with no microscopic junctional activity.[111]

NATURAL FORMATION OF MALIGNANT MELANOMA[22]

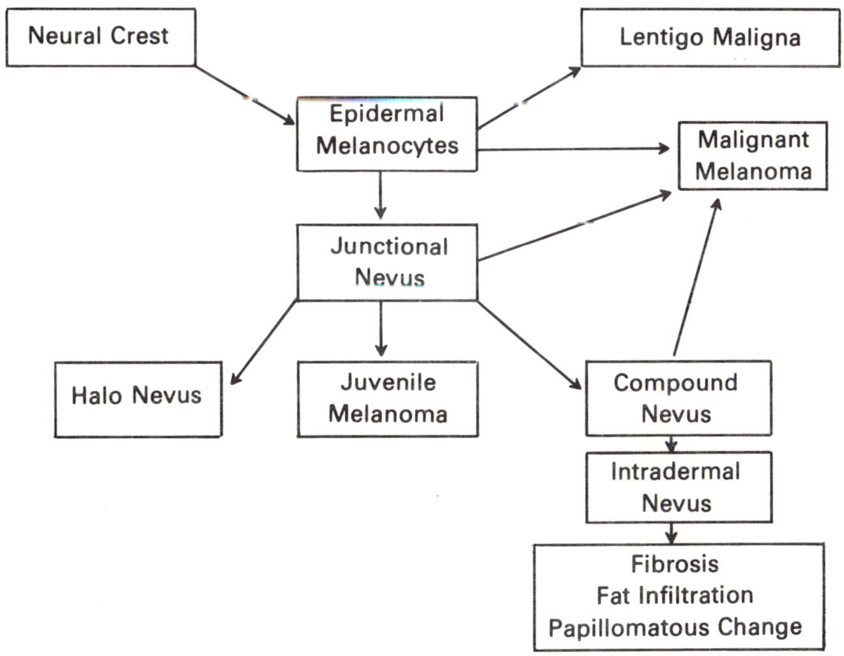

Signs and Symptoms

A patient may present himself with anyone of a myriad of signs or symptoms pertaining to the lesion in question. The suspect lesion may also be an incidental finding on examination.

Change in a lesion in any way is the single most important sign in considering a diagnosis of malignant melanoma. This change can be in size, shape, color, or sensation. Benign nevi seldom change, but its color may get lighter in aging patients and darker in pregnancy.

There are certain types of people and locations that are more commonly associated with malignant melanoma than others. These should be kept in mind and trigger a suspicion.

Race and Complexion: Malignant melanoma ranges from 3.7 to 4.4 cases in the whole population for every one case in negroes.[2 108] Eighty percent of people with malignant melanoma have blonde or red hair, fair skin, blue to green eyes, and tend to freckle when in the sun. These people have very few melanoblasts

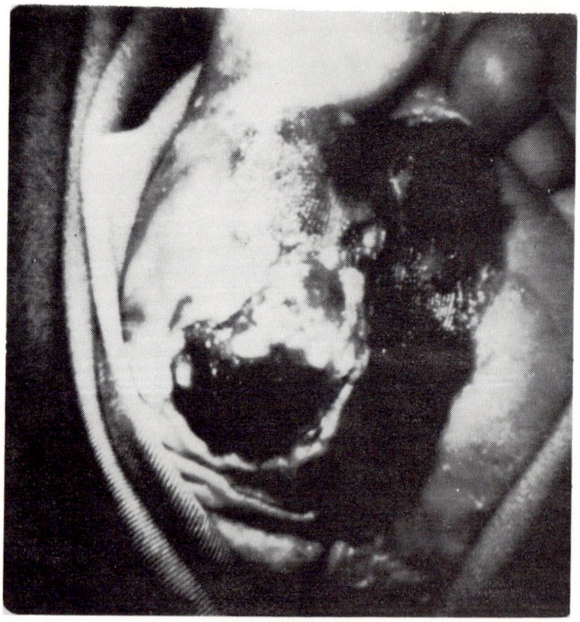

FIGURE 4-6

Large malignant melanoma of the metatarsal region undergoing ulceration and bleeding.

as compared with more darkly skinned people and the melanoblasts tend to be formed in unconcentrated areas.[100] Dark moles in fair people should be excised.[149]

Prepubertal Melanoma: The incidence of melanoma is low until puberty, when there is a sharp rise. From 30-70 years the incidence remains constant. The hormonal changes of puberty make moles that were undetectable, more visable due to an increase in size, pigmentation, and a tendency to elevate above the skin.

Prepubertal or juvenile melanoma is admittedly indistinguishable from malignant melanoma among pathologists unfamiliar with the entity. They are found in children up to puberty and occasionally in young adults. They are benign lesions that are darkly pigmented, blue-black or dark brown, smooth and well demarcated.

Pregnancy: The relationship between melanoma and pregnancy is controversial. Due to the hormonal changes occurring at this time, pigmented areas and nevi tend to become darker in color. There is an estimated three fold increase in the tendency to develop malignant melanoma at this time.[149] Although the cure rate when compared to a non-pregnant person is not effected at comparable stages, the incidence of regional metastasis is doubled. Any pigmented mole in the pregnant female, especially on the palms, soles, or genitalia should be closely watched for change.

Anatomic Location: When compared with the number of benign nevi, there is a greater frequency of melanoma on the soles and genitalia than would be expected. One reason may be the increased number of junctional nevi in these areas and their tendency not to mature into the intradermal type of nevi.

In and around the nail bed, the subungual melanoma or melanotic whitlow is seen more frequently than a benign nevus. It is often confused with a hematoma, chronic paronychia, and subungual keratosis. Many are non-pigmented, unfortunately, but, when present, the pigment may suffuse far beyond the nail bed, producing a characteristic halo of pigment at the top of the digit and down the lateral aspects of the nail surface, which is virtually pathognomonic. Any persistent black lesion involving one nail should be biopsied.[72]

Generally, the regions that tend to have the highest percentage of malignant melanoma when compared to benign nevi, are the soles of the feet, the head and neck, and the genitals. The feet will be dealt with in a separate section.

Those found on the head and neck are usually in elderly persons. They usually begin as a small freckle-like lesion and are non-invasive. They have a good prognosis if removed early, because the tendency for metastasis is not great. This type of melanoma, lentigo maligna melanoma, has a peak age of 70 in caucasians.[28]

Melanomas found on the anogenital area and those of any mucous membrane have a very poor prognosis. These generally begin as junctional nevi and will spread rapidly. Moles in these areas should be excised early.

AGE DISTRIBUTION IN MALIGNANT MELANOMA[149]

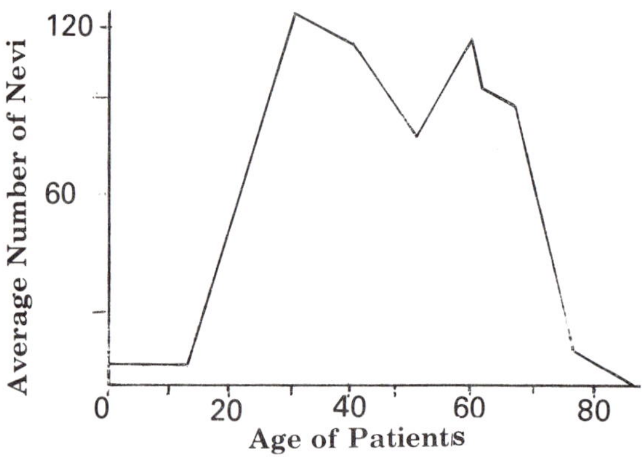

TABLE II
REGIONAL RATIO OF MOLE TO MELANOMA[149]

Moles %	Malignant Melanoma%	Ratio Mole:Melanoma
Head & Neck (13.2	Head & Neck (38.9)	4:9
Upper Extremity (30.2)	Upper Extremity (10.9)	3:1
Trunk (39.3)	Trunk (23.6)	5:3
Genitals (0.1)	Genitals (2.8)	1:28
Lower Extremity (17.2)	Lower Extremity (29.6)	3:5
Soles (.0.2)	Soles (14.5)	1:48

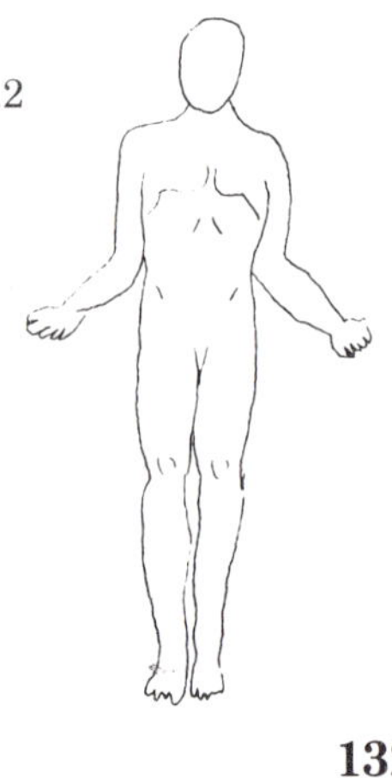

Signs and Symptoms of a Potentially Dangerous Nevus

The patient may relate in a history that an already present nevus has changed in some way. It may have grown in size, changed shape, become darker, or may have just recently appeared. On examination, the color pattern is variegated, the shape has become irregular and it has spread at the borders. This set of circumstances is indication for excision and examination.

Keeping in mind that change is the most important factor, the following is a list of presenting signs in the developing melanoma.[8, 72, 139, 149]

1. Increase in size (diameter or height).
2. Change in surface character.
3. Increase or decrease in the amount of pigment.
4. Spread in a radial manner.
5. Satellite lesions.
6. Scaling.
7. Peeling or exfoliation.
8. Crust formation.
9. Mottling or blotching.
10. Inflammatory areola.
11. Deep brown to black to red halo.
12. Increased vascularity.
13. Localized discomfort or pain.
14. Frog spawn appearance.
15. Itching, prickling, or burning.
16. Ulceration.
17. Bleeding.
18. Serous exudate.
19. Dark or black shiny translucent appearance.
20. Swelling.
21. Bizarre contours.
22. Papillomatous or warty growth.
23. Spontaneous nail avulsion.
24. Regional adenitis.
25. Satellite nodules.
26. Melanuria.

On clinical grounds it is impossible to tell if a mole is a malignant precursor or a malignant melanoma. The signs are many and varied, but all present some sort of change.

Differential Diagnosis

The differential diagnosis for malignant melanoma are many and varied. In 30% — 50% of all cases, the melanoma is preceded by a nevus. It would therefore be of help if the presenting signs could be correlated to a pre-existing nevus. Although the diagnosis of malignant melanoma can only be made after microscopic study, the history can rule out many conditions giving a similar clinical picture.

It is important to keep in mind that the incidence of malignant melanoma in the United States is estimated at 1.8 to 2.6 per 100,000 persons or 1.8 melanomas in 1.5 million nevi.[49 100] They are more common in middle and upper age groups and less common in dark skinned people.

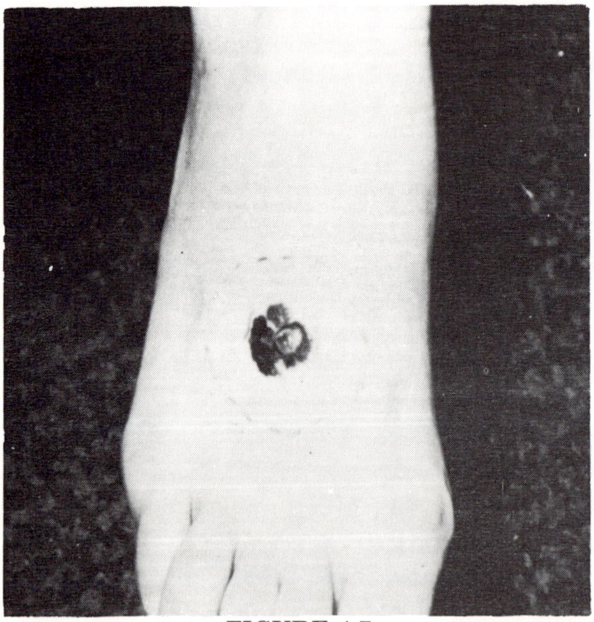

FIGURE 4-7

Malignant melanoma on dorsal aspect of foot revealing central ulcerating area. Outline of surrounding normal skin to be excised with lesion. (Courtesy of Ronald Goldner, M.D., Baltimore, Md.)

Lesions appearing as malignant melanoma clinically are:[8,41,123,149]

1. Benign pigmented nevi.
2. Hutchinson's freckle.
3. Dark hemangiomas.
4. Hemangioepitheliomas.
5. Traumatic blood blisters.
6. Pigmented histiocytomas.
7. Kaposi's sarcoma.
8. Infection underlying a mole.
9. Thrombosed angiokeratomas.
10. Tinea nigra of palms and soles.
11. Accidental pencil lead under the skin.
12. Extra-mammary Paget's disease.
13. Accidental metal incorporation in a benign tumor.
14. Gangrene of finger or toe.
15. Pyogenic granuloma
16. Capillary thrombi and aneurysms.
17. Dark tattoo marks.
18. Pigmented seborrheic keratosis.
19. Minor blood extravasations.
20. Papillary varices.
21. Angiofibromas.
22. Pigmented rodent carcinoma (basal cell and squamous cell).
23. Blue nevi.
24. Juvenile melanoma.
25. Blood cysts.
26. Epidermal inclusion cysts.
27. Giant cell tumor of tendon sheath.
28. Sclerosing hemangiomas.
29. Verruca.
30. Hyperkeratotic lesions.
31. Pigmented areas in Von Recklinghausen's disease.

The diagnosis of a melanotic whitlow or subungal melanoma is also a difficult diagnosis to make. Again, the diagnosis must be made by the pathologist. Due to the position of the nail, it is subject to much trauma and irritation. The history of a preexisting subungual nevus will help in the diagnosis, but there are many conditions to be considered in the differential. Any pigmented lesion associated with the nail and of long time duration

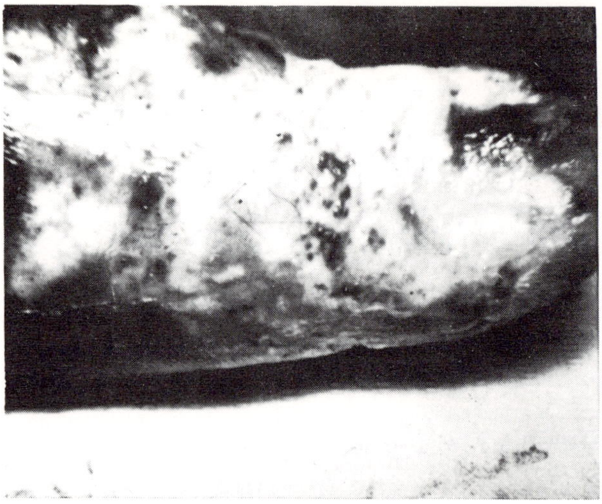

FIGURE 4-8

Melanotic whitlow involving hallux toe revealing black fungating borders.

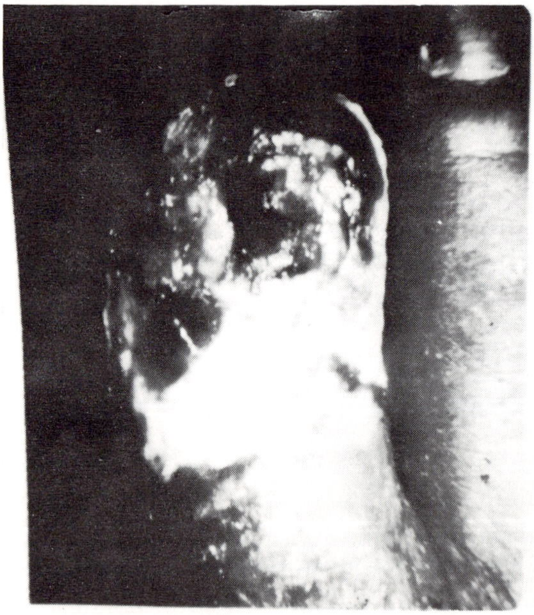

FIGURE 4-9

Malignant melanoma involving hallux toe revealing destruction of surrounding skin. (Courtesy of Leonard Horowitz, D.P.M., Denver, Colorado)

should be biopsied. The following should be considered in the differential diagnosis of melanotic whitlow:

1. Subungual hematoma.
2. Subungual pyogenic granuloma.
3. Subungual pencil lead.
4. Subungual fixed drug reaction.
5. Subungual keratosis.
6. Subungual fibroma.
7. Subungual carcinoma.
8. Metastatic tumor to nail bed.
9. Extragenital chancre.
10. Paronychia.
11. Glomus tumor.
12. Onychomycosis.
13. Gangrene.
14. Subungual Kaposi's sarcoma.

Histology

The microscopic diagnosis of malignant melanoma can be made usually without too much difficulty. The prime characteristic of malignant melanoma is dermal invasion at varying distance from the dermal-epidermal junction. This is usually accompanied by mitotic figures, anaplasia, and an inflammatory infiltrate. The tumor cells are multinucleated, bizarre, giant cells containing varying amounts of melanin pigment. These cells are arranged in loose clusters or poorly defined bundles of fusiform cells. If there are many mitotic figures, anaplasia and melanin pigment, the diagnosis is not too difficult. Stains for activated tyroinase or dihydroxyphenylalanine (dopa) oxidase will usually be positive in melanoma. The tissue specimens must be relatively fresh and unfixed for the stain to take satisfactorily. The special stains are of most value in amelanotic melanoma when melanoma is not suspected clinically. For the purpose of prognosis, the depth of microscopic invasion is used. The more invasion present, the worse the prognosis. The following out line was set up by Clark:[29]

Level I : All tumor cells above basement membrane. By definition, in situ melanoma.

Level II : The neoplastic cells are through the basement membrane extending to the papillary dermis, but not to the reticular dermis. The papillary dermis is the connective tissue layer just below the basement membrane. It is formed of collagen fibers, elastic fibers and ground substance. Melanoma cells found here are evidence of invasion.

Level III: This is an ill-defined area at the interface between the papillary and reticular dermis. It is at this site that the collagen fibers are organizing into bundles. There is no significant invasion into the reticular dermis.

Level IV: The melanoma cells are well into the reticular dermis and are found between the collagen bundles.

Level V : The tumor has invaded into the subcutaneous tissue. Lymphatic or blood vessel invasion, histologically worsens the prognosis.

Any invasion past level III gives a poor prognosis.

Until the microscopic sections are examined by a pathologist, the diagnosis cannot be made. For this reason any suspicious lesion should be examined by excisional biopsy. No suspicious lesion should be treated by destruction because this could result in not identifying the melanoma and grossly undertreating the neoplasm. The ultimate diagnosis rests with the pathologist, and his opinion must be obtained before treating a lesion too lightly, as well as preventing needless radical dissection due to a lesion that clinically resembles melanoma.

Treatment

The prophylactic removal of all nevi is not indicated in the control of malignant melanoma. There are some nevi that deserve special attention and should be watched carefully or prophylactically removed. These include pigmented lesions and nevi with irregular borders, fingerlike projections of pigment or satellite lesions; nevi of nail beds; and dark congenital nevi prior to puberty.[93,149]

The procedure to remove nevi is excisional biopsy. Elliptical incisions following the skin lines should surround the nevus and include normal skin. Subcutaneous tissue should also be removed to allow closure by primary healing. It is not necessary to remove wide margins of skin prior to the pathologist's report. If the pathologist's diagnosis is malignant melanoma, more definitive surgery including radical excision is indicated. Otherwise it is best to leave the patient with a small scar. When a pigmented mole is removed, it never recurs as malignant melanoma.[114]

The therapeutic removal of a malignant melanoma is made by an en bloc, three dimensional removal of tissue including a liberal amount of skin, subcutaneous tissue and fascia.[2,16,43,61,114,119,147] In the foot, when this is not always possible, the treatment should be the removal of a circle of skin 3-5 cm in all directions from the lesion.[49] The defect is closed with a skin graft. A split thickness graft is preferred to a pedicle flap. Closure by first intension has been condemned because of peripheral spread from the primary lesion.[63] Lehman has shown, in a five-year survival rate, that skin grafts give a better result than skin flaps, which in turn give a better result than primary closure.[88] This is possibly due to a host immunity brought with the graft from another site.

Digital melanoma and subungual melanoma are best treated with amputation of the digit at the metatarsal-phalangeal joint or at the tarsal-metatarsal junction.[38,114]

The greatest controversy regarding the treatment of this malignancy is lymph node dissection.[32,58,75,113,114] When melanoma is suspected, it is imperative that the regional lymph nodes be checked. If possible, all nodes in the limb should be examined, ie: the popliteal nodes in the respective fossa and all the inguinal nodes located proximal and distal to the inguinal ligament.[35,58,98,109,114]

When there is lymphadenopathy, the nodes must be dissected. The presence of palpable nodes makes the chance for a complete cure doubtful. Conrad stated that long-term results for patients without node involvement is better than those with involvement.[32] This rationale for lymphadenectomy has led to its routine and wide use. It is the prophylactic removal of nodes, not the therapeutic removal, that is the controversy. Pack feels that this tumor tends to recur locally with such a high frequency, and to metastasize to regional nodes with such a high incidence, that it is imperative for every surgeon treating melanoma to realize the extreme importance of applying radical surgical principles in its care.[114] He is a strong advocate of prophylactic node dissection for any melanoma invading a limb. Gross dissection should be performed before the inguinal nodes are palpable and the procedure can be curative at this stage.[58,98] The groin dissection should be performed about two weeks after the radical excision of the tumor.[88,98] The delay is to allow melanoma cells traveling in the lymphatic vessels time to become embedded in the lymph nodes. It is believed that this would limit regional metastases since the trapped cells are removed. The groin dissection should remove the contents of the femoral triangle, preserving the femoral vessels and nerve, and a lymphadenectomy of the external iliac, obturator and common iliac nodes to the aortic bifurcation. A generous portion of subcutaneous tissue and fascia adjacent to all sides of the femoral triangle are included in an en bloc specimen. A superficial groin dissection omits the pelvic nodes and is limited to the femoral triangle.[45]

McCarthy feels the groin dissection should be limited to those nodes distal to the inguinal ligament.[98] No attempt should be made to include the nodes along the iliac vessels as there were no survivors if the iliac nodes were involved. The dissection of iliac nodes results in a very edematous limb, as there is no lymph flow. Wide excision of the primary site and an incontinuity groin dissection, if feasible, appears to give the patient the best chance for a cure.[45]

The other view is represented by Conrad, where a study of 640 cases showed that wide excision of the primary lesion alone, when compared to wide excision plus lymphadenectomy, had similar figures for survival and recurrence.[32] His theory is that node dissection may cure some patients with positive nodes, but may interfere with a tumor-specific antibody response in others. Lymph nodes should be removed in patients with suspicious nodes and not in those with clinically uninvolved nodes.[32]

Amputation of the limb, disarticulation and quarterectomy should be reserved for cases of local recurrence with node involvement only. In these cases and in cases involving iliac node metastases, the prognosis is very grave. Jones is using a new technique, described by Hueston for patients with regional lymph node and multiple dermal and subcutaneous recurrences, in which he performs a total integumentectomy.[75] He removes skin, subcutaneous tissue and fascia from the entire limb, preserving it as a functional extremity as an alternative to amputation.

In recent years regional chemotherapy has been added to the treatment for melanoma. The suggested procedure is wide local excision, node dissection, and limb isolation perfusion with phenylalanne mustard.[3] The rational according to Creech was to deliver a high dose of cytotoxic agent directly to the tumor and its venous and lymphatic drainage, a dose that would be fatal if administered systemically.[36] Alrich has an 89.5% survival rate with this technique.[3]

At no time should such a lesion be treated by electrodessication, chemical cautery, or radio therapy as total care. If there are no metastases, sharp radical excision of a wide scope may provide a cure. If there is lymphatic spread to nodes, surgery again may allow a cure. However, with a hematogenous spread to the viscera, there is no treatment to save the patient.

Incidence

In a review of the literature the incidence of malignant melanoma involving the lower extremity ranged from 18.0% to 77.7% of the total melanomas. In the foot, the incidence was 3.1 to 41.1% total melanomas.

TABLE III
INCIDENCE OF MALIGNANT MELANONA

	Total Cases	Lower Extremity		Foot	
		Nr.	%	Nr.	%
Charalambidis[25]	250	73	29.2		
Cholnoky[27]	117	30	26.0		
Daland[39]	170	59	30.4	28	16.4
Decker[41]	85	37	40.3	37	40.3
Das Gupta[38]	34	14	41.1	14	41.1
Fortner[45]	220	171	77.7	74	33.6
Hall[62]	222	36	21.9	6	3.1
Lehman[88]	49	9	18.0		
McLeod[99]	498	119	23.9	17	3.4
Meyer[103]	105	34	32.3	19	18.0
Mundth[109]	427	117	27.0		
Pack[117]	862	232	27.0	124	14.4
Pack[116]	1190	360	30.2	142	11.9

Prognosis

There are many factors that alter prognosis. "The typical 'good' tumor has a slow rate of growth, is flat or only slightly raised with a non-ulcerating surface, and has no history of bleeding. It is more often found on the face or leg. Microscopically, there is only slight invasion of the dermis. The prognosis is good, and over 80% survive five years. The typical 'bad' tumor is quite different. It is more often found on the trunk though it may occur anywhere. It is faster growing, raised, ulcerating, and sometimes non-pigmented. Microscopically, there is often invasion of the dermal lymphatics. . . ."[14]

The ten year survival of 150 consecutive cases of malignant melanoma studied by Bodenham is just under 40%. Females have a 10% to 15% advantage over males. Most of the deaths occur in the first four years. The average five year survival rate is just over 50%.[14]

TABLE IV
FIVE-YEAR SURVIVAL RATE ACCORDING TO LOCATION ON THE LOWER LIMBS

	Location	Nr. Cases	Nr. Survived	%Survived
Pack[116]	subungual	24	7	38.9
	leg	125	30	30.6
	foot	59	15	31.2
Mundth[109]	leg	89	43	48.0
Watson[146]	foot & toes	40	20	50.0
	ankle	17	12	70.6
Lehman[88]	leg	9	4	44.4
Fortner[45]	leg	54	21	38.9
	foot	54	14	25.9
	toes	20	6	30.0
Charalambidis[25]	leg	65	25	38.5

Fortner believes the prognosis is worse in the toes and feet than when the lesion is in the leg and thigh.[45] It does appear that lesions on the hands, feet, and mucous membranes have a poorer prognosis than when found in other places.[16,45,84,109]

Age is significant in the prognosis. Melanoma capable of metastasis are rare in children. Time may be the most important factor. "Patients who obtain early, adequate treatment of melanoma have a remarkably good prognosis."[25] For this reason, women have a better prognosis then men, ie: women are more concerned with blemishes than men, and will generally seek help sooner. Melanoma in women also tend to be more superficial and their resistance to melanoma growth is better than in men.[2,45,109] Generally, the survival rate for women is 10% better than in men if there are no positive lymph nodes.[45]

With invasion of lymph nodes the prognosis drops drastically. This tumor can metastasize through the lymph channels or through hematogenous spread. The most common type of spread is to the regional lymph nodes. At this point a cure is still possible through node dissection and limb perfusion, but prognosis is not favorable. Spread through the hematogenous route gives a very grave prognosis because the tumor can spread to any part of the body.

The size of the lesion is significant in terms of prognosis. Tumors less than 2 cm. in diameter carry a good prognosis. Depth of the lesion is very important, as reviewed in Clark's classification.[29]

Surprisingly enough, there are cases of spontaneous regression mentioned in the literature.[14] This is by far the exception. It is disturbing that . ."in a surprisingly high percentage of cases, five year survival of a malignant melanoma exhibits a diathesis for the activation of junctional nevi in various parts of the body, but particularly in the vicinity of the primary tumor. The phenomenon, called satellitosis, carries a poor prognosis and is seen in 19 to 25% of cases involving the foot after groin dissection.[16,140]

Ulceration and/or bleeding of any size lesion is a poor prognostic sign, unless it is caused by trauma, in which case it would be misleading.[49,143] Clinical and microscopic involvement of the regional lymph nodes has a very bad prognosis.

Olsen has clinically staged the tumor as follows:[113]

1. No clinical signs of metastasis.
2. Clinically enlarged and suspicious regional lymph nodes and/or a few cutaneous metastases close to the primary tumor (satellites).
3. Other signs of metastases, ie, further groups of lymph nodes, cutaneous satellites along the lymphatic trunk, remote whenever metastases and visceral metastases.

The best chance for a cure comes with early detection and adequate surgical treatment. Proper examination, awareness, and high clinical suspicion are the best tools to fight this problem.

Basal Cell Carcinoma
(Basal Cell Epitheloma)

INTRODUCTION

Basal cell carcinoma (BCC) is an epithelial skin neoplasm originating from the epidermal basal layer. An impaired ability of basal cells to mature and keratinize accounts for the tumor development. This impairment prevents the cells from being shed during the normal keratinizing process.[7, 91, 107] Basal cell carcinoma is the most common skin cancer and potentially the most curable. It comprises about 80% of all skin cancers; it rarely metastasizes and the "cure rate" (complete arrest of growth of tumor cells) can be 100% if found early and treated adequately. Metastatic exceptions have been reported (Binkley and Rauschkalb).[11] Sauer thinks that metastasizing basal cell epithelioma probably represents a wrong diagnosis.[129] Death from basal cell carcinoma usually results from neglect on the part of the patient in not seeking professional advice soon enough.

The occurrence in adults is much more common than in children, being most frequently seen in male patients above the age of 50.

The term epithelioma is used by many authors as a synonym for carcinoma. Becker suggested the term epithelioma should be used for benign epidermal tumors and the term carcinoma for malignant epidermal tumors.[5]

Etiology

1. *External initiating Agent* — The major external agent for BCC is ultraviolet light (2000-7200 A). It acts as an agent that starts the first essential phase predisposing to the occurrence of BCC. These rays are absorbed by both the epidermis and the dermis and stimulation toward neoplasm depends on the cummulative effects of repeated exposures, not an isolated episode of intense exposure.[102] There is much conflicting information about the action responsible for cutaneous reaction to ultra violet light,

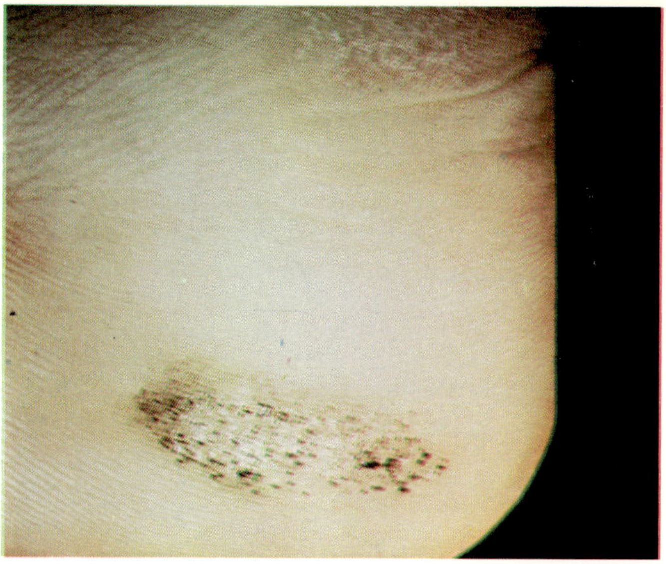

Black Heel — Often confused with mosiac warts. Can occur over any area from repeated pressure and friction. (Courtesy Ronald Goldner, M.D., Baltimore, Maryland.)

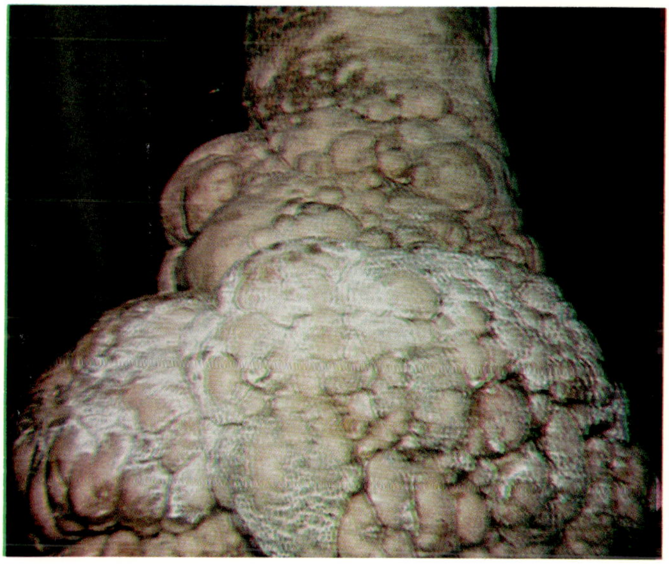

Elephantiasis Nostras Verrucosa — Presenting as a severe verrucous type deformity of the foot. (Courtesy of Howard Imanuel, D.P.M. Ft. Myers, Florida.

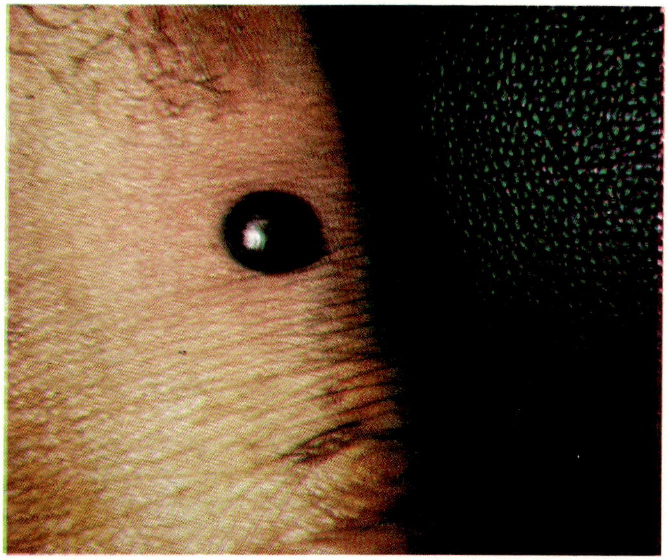

Histocytoma — Usually firm, button type lesions. These lesions are dark in color due to amounts of hemosiderin and lipid deposits. (Courtesy of Richard Gibbs, M.D., New York City, N.Y.)

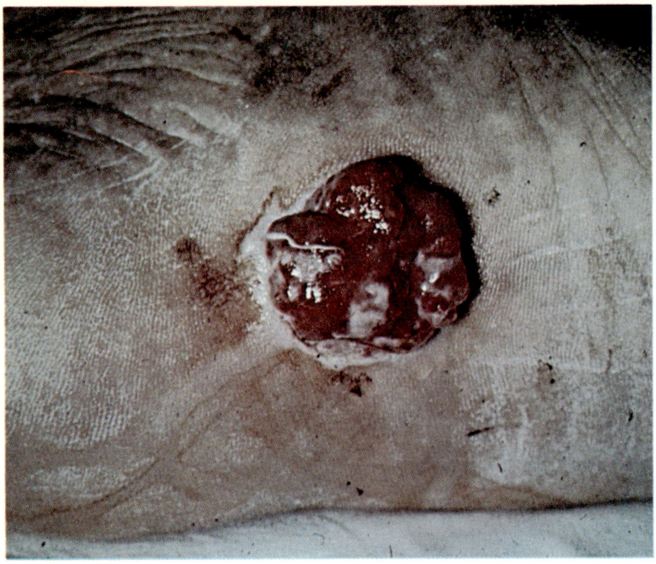

Eccrine Poroma — This is a benign tumor usually occuring as a solitary lesion on the sole in patients past 40. It appears sessile or slightly pedunculated, has a normal or erythematous color and has a firm rubbery consistency. Ulceration may occur at points of pressure, but the surface is usually smooth or lobulated. Differential diagnosis: granuloma pyogenicum, amelanotic melanoma, keloid, squamous cell carcinoma. Courtesy of William V. R. Shellow, M.D., Los Angeles, California.)

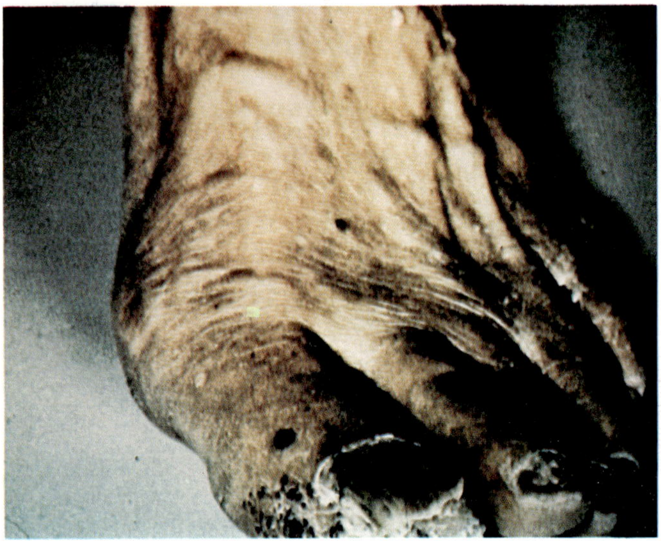

Angiokeratoma Mibelli — Dark red to purplish papules in color and may have a verrucous or hyperkeratotic surface. (Courtesy of James Ganley, D.P.M., Norristown, Pa.)

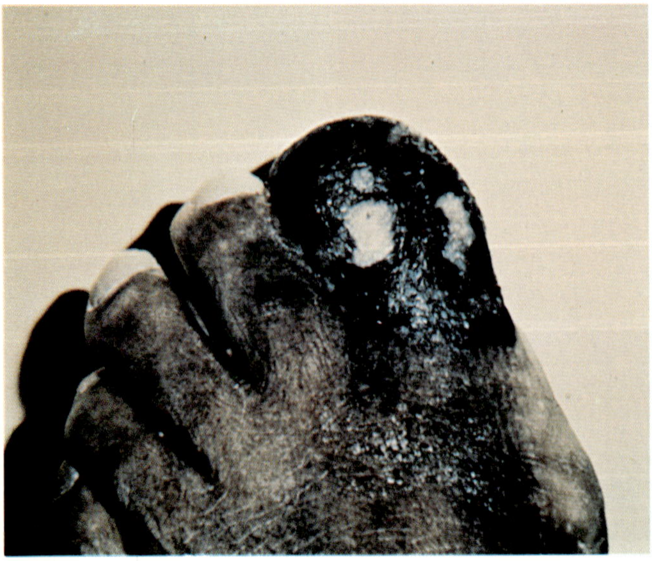

"Malignant" Lentigo Maligna Melanoma — Usually a slow developing from of melanoma, rarely seen on the foot. Differential diagnosis: Gangrene with involving digit. Most commonly seen exposed surfaces such as the face.

though the etiologic role of ultra violet light in regard to BCC is generally not disputed.[102]

2. *Predisposing Factors* — Blond, light complexioned individuals are particularly vulnerable. (Occupations in which people are under continuous solar exposure, such as farming, sailing, and sports, are particularly hazardous).

Histopathology

The characteristic cell of basal cell epithelioma (basalioma cell) is a cell with a large, oval nucleus containing little cytoplasm. Although the nuclei resemble closely those of the epidermal basal cell layer, the basalioma cell differs from basal cells by not showing intercellular bridges on light microscopy (Lever).[91] The nuclei, as a rule, have a rather uniform appearance rather than an anaplastic picture. Thus, little pronounced variation in size or intensity, and no abnormal mitosis, even in rare cases of BCC with metastases, is seen.

Histologically, basal cell carcinoma can be divided into two groups; undifferentiated and differentiated. Differentiation toward the cutaneous appendages (hair, sebeceous, apocrine or eccrine glands) is characteristic of the differentiated group. Basal cell carcinoma showing no differentiation are called solid basal cell epithelioma; those differentiating toward hair structures are called keratotic; toward sebaceous glands, cystic; toward apocrine or eccrine glands, adenoid basal cell carcinoma. Types of basal cell carcinoma which may be seen on the pedal surfaces:

1. *Nodulo-ulcerative type of basal cell carcinoma* — This type may show either differentiation or no differentiation. The solid, differentiated BCC has tumor masses of various sizes and shapes in the dermis. The keratotic, cystic and adenoid BCC have a characteristic histologic appearance depending on what cutaneous appendage they differentiate to.

2. *Pigmented BCC* — This type usually shows little or no differentiation (solid BCC). The presence of melanin can be explained by the fact that melanocytes are present both in the surface epidermis and the primary epithelial germ cells.

3. *Sclerosing BCC (Morphea-like)* — This type shows little or no differentiation (solid BCC). This varient shows connective tissue proliferation to a much greater extent than the other types of BCC.

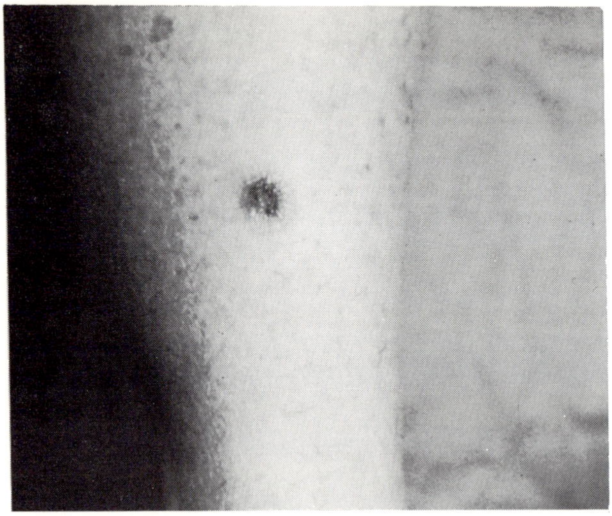

FIGURE 4-10

Basal cell carcinoma involving posterior surface o' lower leg. This lesion is undergoing ulcerative changes. (Courtesy of Richard Gibbs, M.D., N.Y., New York)

4. *Superficial BCC* — This also is basically a solid type of BCC with irregular proliferations and buds of tumor attached to the epidermis (often multicentric).

Sites of Predilection

BCC is found almost exclusively on the face and head and less frequently on other hair-bearing skin (trunk). The periorbital region of the face is by far the most common site — the site most easily exposed to the sun.

Clinical Picture

1. Nodulo-ulcerative (Rodent-ulcer) — This is the most common type of BCC beginning as a firm, non-inflammatory, indolent, waxy papule or nodule. This small waxy papule often shows small telangiectatic vessels on the surface that slowly enlarge over the years, then develop a central ulceration surrounded by a pearly border. This end stage is called the "rodent-ulcer." Hence, nodulo-ulcerative BCC is a slow growing, locally destructive neo-

plasm most often occuring in middle-aged men; the face is most often involved.

2. Pigmented BCC — differs from the nodulo-ulcerative type only by the addition of brown or black pigmentation.

3. Sclerosing BCC — This uncommon type of BCC manifests as a minimally elevated, firm white or yellowish plaque with an ill-defined border, which rarely undergoes ulceration.

4. Superficial BCC — This manifests as a single or multiple reddish, scaly, slightly infiltrated patch with fine hair-like borders. Commonly seen on the trunk whereas the previous variants are seen most on the face and neck.

5. Others — Premalignant fibroepithelioma BCE, nevoid BCE syndrome, linear basal cell nevus.

Natural History

BCC grows slowly over a period of years, but rapid growth periods do occur. Destructive invasion of local tissues, such as bone, cartilage and other skin areas, cause serious morbidity and mortality, if neglected; secondary infection with pain can then occur.

Diagnosis

1. *History* — The only reasonable early sign of BCC is the patient feeling a firm, raised papule in the skin. Any superficial crusted ulcer which has not healed over a period of months should be investigated. Trauma may also be an etiologic agent, but any scarred area may be considered a predisposed site.

The pearly raised border with a central ulceration is highly characteristic of BCC. Radiographic films and laboratory studies play no helpful part in the diagnosis.

2. *Biopsy* — Biopsy must always be performed since no clinician's judgement is infallible (15-20% error among experts). This especially holds for foot lesions, since BCC on the sole does not have a characteristic clinical or histologic appearance.

Differential Diagnosis

The multiplicity of skin lesions mimicking BCC is highly varied. Simple biopsy will usually distinguish one from the other and it should be employed both for the patient's welfare and the clinicans education. Some of the more common lesions that must be distinguished from BCC are:

1. Pyogenic granuloma — soft lesion of recent onset.
2. Sclerosing hemangioma — hard, pigmented lesion, usually on thighs and legs.
3. Seborrheic keratosis — greasy, soft, pigmented and warty.
4. Psoriasis — flat, scaly, on extensor limb surfaces.
5. Squamous cell carcinoma — more rapid growth than BCC, more inflammation, firm, scaly papule with no pearly telangiectatic border.
6. Cavernous hemangioma — bluish, soft and compressible.
7. Keratoacanthoma — affects same areas as BCC, but is rapidly growing and in a few weeks, involutes spontaneously.
8. Other skin lesions: adnexal tumors, metastatic cancer, sebaceous adenoma, warts, nevi, small cysts, melanoma, and scars from previous injury or radiation.

Basal cell carcinoma involving the dorsal surfaces of the pedal skin are more readily recognized than lesions of the sole. Nodular-ulcerative forms, however, can be confused with amelanotic melanoma, where the pigmented variety may be confused with malignant melanoma, seborrheic keratosis and verruca. Basal cell carcinoma of the sole progresses slowly ranging from 2-30 years and is difficult to diagnose clinically in this location, since it takes on an atypical appearance. This lesion may even present itself as a scaly, granulomatous keratotic, or eroded area suggesting even an eccrine poroma or plantar callous.

Pedal Involvement

Basal cell carcinoma (BCC) occuring on the foot is extremely rare, but cases have been reported. Their appearance on nonglabrous skin has stimulated controversy as to its postulated histogenesis. One theory is the primary epithelial germ cell development of BCC. These are immature, pluripotential cells with a tendency to differentiate toward hair follicles, apocrine and sebaceous glands.[91] Since the plantar surface of the foot contains none of these structures, the consensus is that BCC arising in this area cannot derive from cells analogous to primary epithelial germ cells.

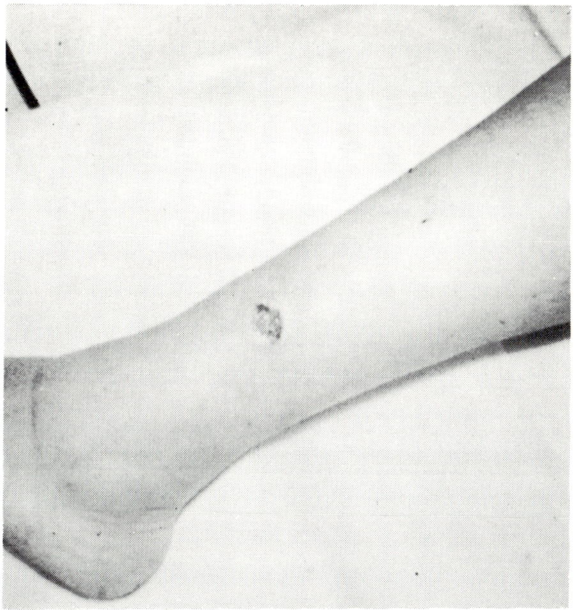

FIGURE 4-11

Basal cell carcinoma above lateral malleolus. The lesion is deeply ulcerated and does not respond to conservative care. (Courtesy of Isidore Zeligman, M.D., Baltimore, Md.)

A second postulated theory of BCC histogenesis takes into consideration the pluripotentiality of epidermal cells. Whether or not immature cells with the potential of forming eccrine sweat glands can give rise to BCC has been uncertain. Eccrine sweat gland germ cells arise somewhat later in intrauterine life than primary epithelial germ cells. Eccrine sweat glands are plentiful on the sole; consequently, BCC of the sole probably arises from cells analgous to eccrine sweat gland germ cells.[95] Such a concept simply broadens the theoretical histogenesis of BCC to embrace not only cells analgous to primary epithelial germ cells, but also to eccrine sweat gland germ cells. "It may be more accurate to state that BCE derived from immature pluripotential epithelial cells, which normally differentiate into any of the epithelial structures of the skin."[95]

The first reported case of BCC on the foot was by Schreiner and Wehr (1933).[131] Their case was one out of 37 primary malignant foot tumors; they included neither illustrations nor histologic details of the lesion. It was treated with radium and said to have resulted in a cure. Since it was radiosensitive, various authors (Hyman and Michaelides; Lewis et al) contend it was probably BCC of an undifferentiated type rather than eccrine poroma, which is radioresistant.[71,95]

One series reported by Sachs and Garbe (1937) contained no references to a BCC of the soles (or palms)[128], but Zugerman (1957) learned that Sachs has since encountered six cases of BCC of the sole.[153]

Pascher and Sims (1954) reported two cases of BCC, undifferentiated type, of the sole.[118] In neither case was the diagnosis made on clinical differential. This is understandable in view of the usual site and atypical appearance of many skin lesions on the plantar aspect of the foot. Biopsy and histologic examination assured the diagnosis in both cases.

Zugerman (1957) reported two cases of BCC of the sole.[153] In

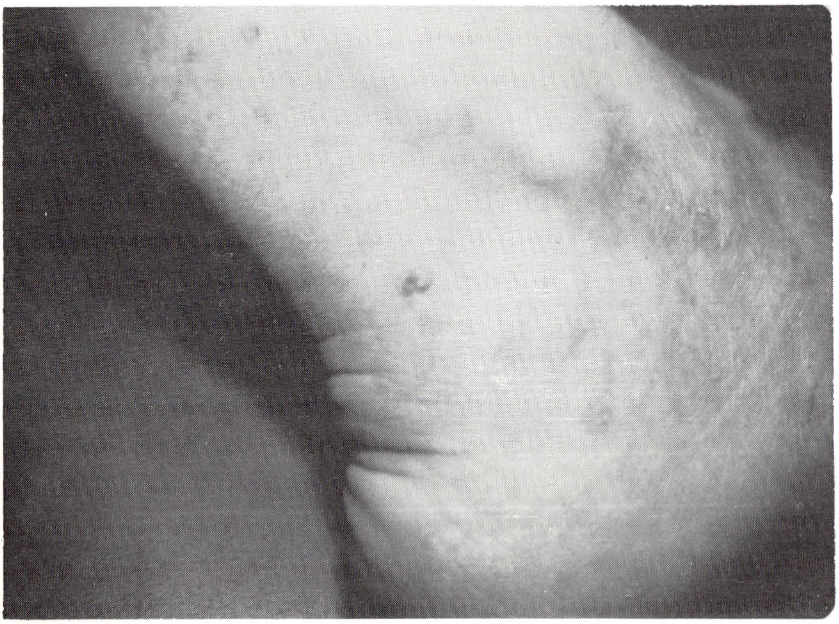

FIGURE 4-12

Basal cell and Bowen's disease of ankle due to arsenic. (Courtesy of Richard Gibbs, M.D., New York, New York)

one of the two cases, the epithelioma arose "probably from the sweat duct as a syringoma."[153] Some authors, (Hyman and Michaelides, Okun et al),[71,111] after examining the photomicrographs in Zugerman's paper, think that both lesions were actually eccrine poromas, rather than BCC. Pinkus et al (1956), made a significant report of foot lesions in five patients which were called "eccrine poromas."[122] These lesions arise from the intraepidermal portion of the sweat duct or acrosyringum. Zugerman's first case was a 67 year old white female complaining of a painful growth on the ball of the left foot.[153] She had been treated for a plantar wart with no relief. The growth had been present for seven years, and except for pain due to pressure, no unusual signs or symptoms were noted. Examination revealed a dry, dusky red, granulomatous tumor, with a sharp, nonpearly edge measuring 1.5 cm. in diameter. It was situated on the sole below the fourth toe. Treatment consisted of local excision. Zugerman's second case was a 42 year old male presenting with a benign appearing, skin colored, painless, fleshy growth on the plantar surface of the medial longitudinal arch of the left foot. The tumor was 3 cm. in diameter and showed no evidence of previous ulceration. The case responded in a similar fashion to the first one.

Hunter and Hollier (1960) reported BCC of the sole in one patient which, on histologic examination, was first thought to be BCC, but later it was thought to be similar to an eccrine poroma and should be considered a form of BCC or as a separate entity. They concluded that the cases of Pinkus et al (1956) and their own should be differentiated from BCC and hence be considered a separate entity.[121]

Hyman and Michaelides (1963) reported a unique case of the fibroepithelial type of BCC on the sole.[71] This is the first reported case of this type of BCC on the sole. These authors believe that some of the cases of BCC of the sole are indeed eccrine poromas (Pinkus et al, 1956).[122] The histologic features of their case were consistent with the "fibroepithelial tumor of Pinkus" (1953) variety of BCC.[121]

Lewis et al (1956) reported a case of BCC of the sole in which a 36 year old female, former X-ray technician, with previous breast carcinoma, was seen with cutaneous lesions of the right temple left shoulder, and left submandibular area.[95] The lesions were present for three years and after histologic examination, a superficial BCC was diagnosed. Four months later, a lesion was present on the right plantar surface of the third metatarsal head. The lesion was 1 cm, slightly indurated and covered by a firmly adherent scale. Histologic examination proved to be a superficial BCC. Recurrence was noted eight months later when a wide excision was performed. The histologic picture was again characteristic of BCC. This appears to be a unique case of the superficial type of BCC on the sole.

Berger et al (1966) reported a case of BCC of the sole which was of the premalignant fibroepithelial type (Pinkus-1953).[9,121] It occurred in a 63 year old white female who had a previous history of multiple BCC on the head, a very common site. Examination revealed a lesion 4 mm in diameter, sharply demarcated, elevated, brown-orange nodule in the midportion of the left sole. The lesion was neither painful nor tender. The initial clinical diagnosis was plantar verruca, but BCC was considered due to the unusual color and fleshy nodular consistency.

Gold (1967) reported a case of BCC of the sole on a 47 year old negro female.[55] The lesion was on the plantar-medial arch area of the sole. Examination revealed a nodular, elevated, shiny lesion, measuring 1/2 cm by 3/4 cm, oval in shape, salmon-reddish color, showing some telangiectatic vessels. Surgical excision and histologic examination was reported as BCC.

Weitzner (1968) reported the first case of BCC involving the web of the toes.[148] His communication with Pinkus and Zackheim was note worthy since neither had encountered BCC in the digital interphalangeal skin before. Weitzner reported that in seven cases of BCC by previous researchers, he found only one BCC of the combined 5,509 lesions on the foot (Schrek, 1941),[132] and its exact location was not revealed. The case by Weitzner was a 50 year old Spanish-American man who presented with what was thought to be a junctional neuvs. The patient had a previous BCC on the nose six years before the plantar lesion. It was described as a 4x4 mm flat, black area in the web of the right second and third toes. The lesion was excised with the clinical diagnosis of junctional nevus. The operative site healed without complication, and no recurrence or new lesion has occurred. Histologic examination revealed a pigmented BCC.

Treatment

Local wide excision can be used in slow-growing, localized BCC. A margin of one cm suffices for most small lesions. Surgery offers a curative method of treatment when skillfully applied. Cosmetic results should be taken into account since the cure rate is high. Curettage followed by electrodessiccation or radiation is widely used by dermatologists. Mohs' chemosurgery is a recognized form of treatment in special cases. However, the technique is specialized and requires study, training, and clinical skill in order to judge the depth of the lesion.

Pathologic studies of skin margins should be a rule in surgical excision. Surgical excision of a BCC is the only method of treatment that should be attempted by those who only occasionally are exposed to this neoplasm.

To surgically excise the lesion, the following procedures should be employed:

1. Anesthetize the area.
2. Make an elliptical incision with the scalpel to include at least 2 to 5 mm around the borders.
3. Close the incision (skin grafting may be necessary).

If the pathologist states that the tumor extended up to the edge of the excision, a further, more radical excision may be required. Have the patient return for periodic check-ups in one month, two months, and three months, then yearly for 3-5 years. This treatment procedure is mainly for the nodulo-ulcerative or pigmented types of BCC.

Treatment of deeply ulcerated lesions, fibrosing or superficial BCC should come within the domain of the dermatologist, surgeon, and radiologist. When the rodent ulcer has a deep ulceration, surgical excision is questionable especially if local, destructive changes of bone or cartilage have occurred.

Common Errors

Ackerman and del Regato list some factors, in order of importance, that contribute to failure to cure skin cancer in general:[1]

1. Little or no skill by treating physician.
2. Use of single method for all lesions.
3. Lack of pathologic control of margins.
4. Lack of post-treatment study of suspicious areas.
5. Failure to receive careful follow-up.

Prognosis

The outlook for absolute cure of BCC is excellent. No one need die of BCC. They cause death where there is inadequate treatment or neglect, thereby allowing the neoplasm to recur and invade surrounding structures.

Squamous Cell Carcinoma (Prickle Cell Carcinoma, Epidermoid Carcinoma)

INTRODUCTION

Squamous cell carcinoma is a malignant neoplasm of epidermal origin. Squamous cell carcinoma of the extremities are infrequent tumors, the literature being inconsistent with regards to prognosis and etiology.[53] They comprise not more than 1% of all primary carcinomas in different parts of the body.[24] Although amenable to early diagnosis and definitive forms of treatment, squamous cell carcinoma of the extremities is often treated as a benign lesion for long periods of time without biopsy.

This neoplasm of the skin, in general, is regarded as one of the undesired effects of extensive exposure to sunlight. This chapter will focus on the other predisposing factors leading to squamous cell carcinoma of the extremities. These include mechanical, chemical and thermal changes and the various organic skin changes found in association with this tumor.

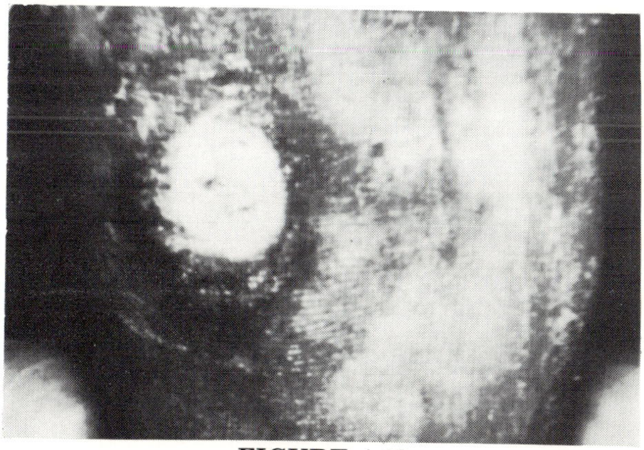

FIGURE 4-13

Squamous cell carcinoma of heel revealing irregular pattern of central ulceration. (Courtesy of Sanford Rosenfeld, D.P.M., Detroit, Michigan)

Etiology

The following is a brief discussion of the predisposing causes that appear to be related to the general occurrence of squamous cell carcinoma.

1. Ultra-violet sunlight
   The lesions are common on exposed parts of the body and occur frequently in persons exposed to sunlight.[13] Sun-damaged skin, due to prolonged exposure to ultra-violet light and/or inadequate protection against the sun's rays, are responsible for the majority of these tumors.[91]
2. Ionizing radiation
   The lesions may occur in areas subjected to prolonged and/or severe radiation.
3. Chronic irritation
   Squamous cell carcinoma secondary to pre-existing skin lesions are uncommon, but by no means rare. The majority of antecedent lesions occuring before squamous lesions develop are:
   a. Old burn scars[19]
   b. Chronic osteomyelitic sinuses[34]
   c. Stasis ulcers[42]

   The low incidence of squamous cell carcinoma on the foot, either as a primary lesion or secondary to some organic skin lesion, approximately 1.5% of all squamous carcinomas, suggests that the constant trauma of walking, which often leads to pressure plantar callosities under metatarsal heads, may not, by itself, be a prime factor in the carcinogenesis.[64,90]

   Bick (1932) stated that the relationship of malignancy to the presence of trauma or chronic irritation is striking.[10] Taylor, et al, (1941) showed 193 cases (45% of all the cases) in which there were precancerous lesions.[41] The distribution was as follows:

   63 — pre-existing keratosis
   36 — old injury and scar
   23 — old burn scar
   14 — arsenical keratosis
   11 — osteomyelitic sinus
   13 — associated with varicose ulcers
   10 — previous irradiation dermatitis

4 — tar dermatitis
19 — misc. lesions.
DeBell and Stevenson (1936) pointed out that Marjolin, in 1828, emphasized that skin epithelioma frequently develop in sites of old scars.[40] Epitheliomas developing on old burn scars have been named "Marjolin's ulcer". Broders (1921) found about 52% of his cases of epithelioma in all parts of the body were preceded by a pre-existing lesion. A history of injury was elicited in approximately 24% of the cases.[20] Squamous cell carcinoma arising in chronic osteomyelitic foci is uncommon although well documented. Sedlin and Fleming (1963) reported 71 cases developing at these sites. A rate of 31% were found to metastasize.[134]

4. Carcinogenic hydrocarbons
   Lesions were formerly common on the scrotum of chimney sweeps and on the skin of mule skinners who worked with oils that soaked into their clothes. Pitch, tar and paraffin also have carcinogenic compounds.
5. Arsenic
   Lesions are common in industrial workers and others exposed to arsenical pesticides.
6. Others
   Squamous cell carcinoma have also occurred in lesions of chronic discoid lupus enythematosis and lupus vulgaris.

Classification Based on Source

Volkman's original classification, used in 1889, for squamous carcinomas of the extremities is still a useful tool.[22 76] It is divided into three main groups:

1. Those developing in chronic inflammatory tissue (infection, scar, irritation, trauma)
2. Those developing from some previous neoplasm
3. Those developing on apparently normal skin

Clinical Picture

The lesion begins most commonly in its primary form as a superficial, scaly, slightly indurated maculopapule which bleeds and resists casual therapy. Later, a shallow ulcer central to the lesion, surrounded by a thick, wide, elevated and indurated border usually appears.[91] The lesion will not heal spontaneously, nor respond to other prescribed therapy usually given in early, unrecognized cases.

The ulcer may be covered by a crust concealing a red, pseudogranular base. The ulcerative stage is usually reached in a few months, but may take several years. Occasionally, raised, fungoid, verrucous lesions without ulceration may also be seen.

Diagnosis

An adequate history is essential for the diagnosis. Early symptoms may be the feeling of a firm, raised skin nodule, or perhaps an area of thickening in previously normal skin. Increase in pain and drainage from chronic benign lesions should suggest the development of malignant lesions.

A biopsy of any ulceration other than ischemic ulcerations of the lower extremity should be an intergal part of the diagnostic examination before any form of excisional therapy is planned.[150]

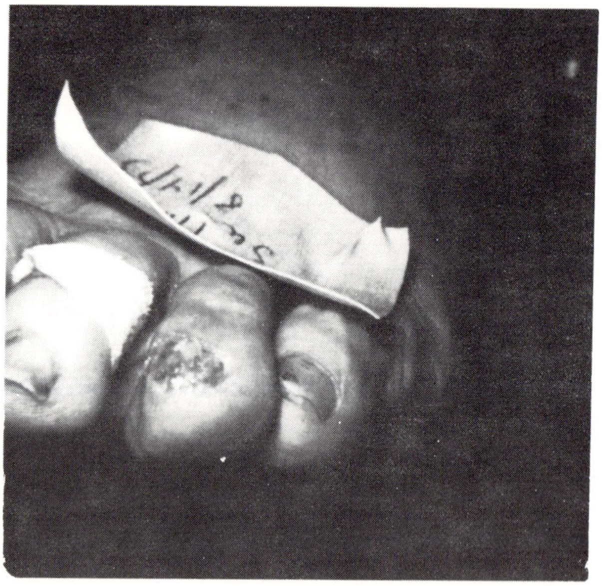

FIGURE 4-14

Squamous cell carcinoma of nail bed. Previous history of chronic paronychia. No bone involvement was present.

Differential Diagnosis

The histological diagnosis is easily made in typical cases, but may be difficult at times. It must be differentiated from solar keratosis, keratoacanthoma and basal cell epithelioma, both histologically and clinically.

The difference between squamous carcinoma and solar keratosis is in the degree rather than in the type of changes. In squamous carcinoma actual invasion of the dermis is present and the invading tumor mass may contain horn pearls. No sharp line exists between the two conditions, and it is not infrequent to find confusion between the two.[91] Solar keratosis can be said to represent squamous cell carcinoma, grade one-half. Solar keratosis also occurs at similar sites as squamous cell carcinoma. The lesions are usually less than 1 cm in diameter, have dry, hard scales which are firmly adherent to an erythematous base and occasionally shows marked hyperkeratosis.

Localized keratoacanthoma, in the early stages, is difficult, and at times impossible to distinguish from squamous cell carcinoma. Unless an elliptical specimen from the center of the lesion is excised including the edge on both sides, diagnosis may be very hard. The most important diagnostic feature aside from the structure, is the high degree of keratinization manifested by an eosinophilic, glossy cellular appearance. Clinical data is also of great aid, for it usually occurs as a solitary, hemispheric nodule, one cm in diameter. The nodule reaches its full size in a few weeks, and involutes spontaneously within a few months. Rapid growth and the appearance of a horn-filled crater will also help specify keratoacanthoma. Healing takes place with a slightly depressed scar. In case of doubt, it is best to consider the lesion as a squamous cell carcinoma and procede on that basis.

Differentiation of basal cell epithelioma from squamous cell carcinoma is often difficult. An intermediary form called basal-squamous cell epithelioma exists. However, as a rule, differentiation is fairly easy. Most cells of basal epithelioma stain deeply basophilic, whereas most cells of squamous carcinoma stain eosinophilic if they are grade one or two. Grade three or four show basophilic stain but also show greater atypical cells than basal cell epithelioma. Basal cell carcinoma is also a slow growing tumor and shows pearly, telangiectatic borders with a central ulceration.

Histopathology

Squamous cell carcinoma is a true invasive surface epidermal carcinoma. The anaplastic squamous cells invade irregularly from the epidermal layer in sheets into the dermis.[91] The invading masses are composed of differentiated squamous and horny cells and of differentiated (anaplastic, atypical) squamous cells. The greater the number of atypical squamous cells, the more malignant the tumor. Differentiation is in the direction of keratinization. Horn cells are characteristic structures composed of concentric layers of squamous cells having gradually increasing keratinization toward the center.

Broders (1921) introduced a system of grading squamous cell carcinoma.[20] He set up four grades according to the proportion of differentiated cells to undifferentiated and atypical cells.

Grade I - more than 75% of cells differentiated
Grade II - more than 50% of cells differentiated
Grade III - more than 25% of cells differentiated
Grade IV - less than 25% of cells differentiated

Since differentiation is in the direction of keratinization, it represents the essential features of the Broders grading system. Depth of penetration of the lesion is also very important. Lesions remaining locally malignant are not usually grade I or II; after ulceration, there is usually early metastasis revealing grade III or IV.

Bone Involvement

Destruction of bone in squamous cell carcinoma secondary to chronic osteomyelitis is due largely to bacterial infection, rather than neoplastic invasion.[24] The invading bacteria is thought to breakdown the natural barrier and allow the neoplasm to enter as a secondary invader. The necrotic bone is then replaced with neoplastic bone. The complete eradication of osteomyelitic foci with modern surgical techniques combined with antibiotics may greatley reduce the number of possible squamous cell carcinomas at these sites.[76] Chronic nail infections could easily involve the bone in the foot. The authors have recently experienced such a case.

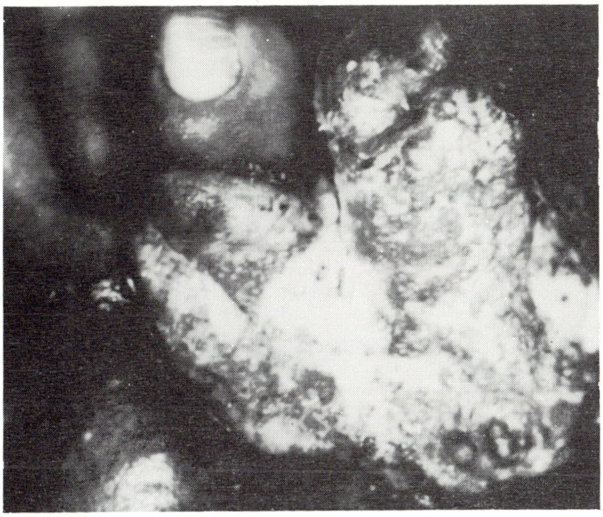

FIGURE 4-15

Squamous cell carcinoma involving 4th & 5th digits. (Courtesy of Leon Cohen, D.P.M., Carlsbad, N.M.)

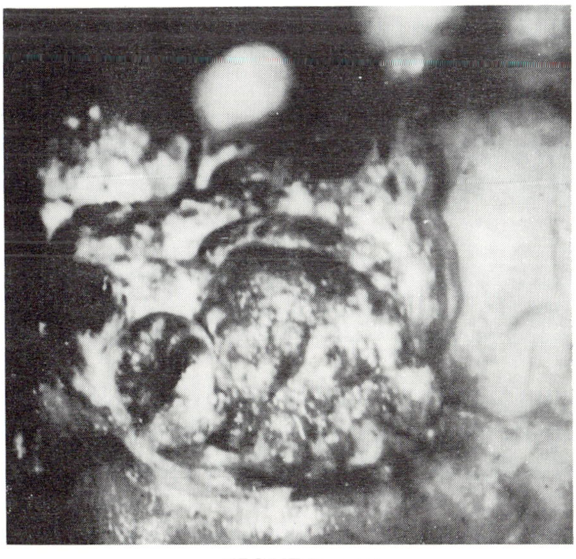

FIGURE 4-16

Complete destruction from squamous cell penetrating dorsal and plantar skin surfaces. (Courtesy of Leon Cohen, D.P.M., Carlsbad, N.M.)

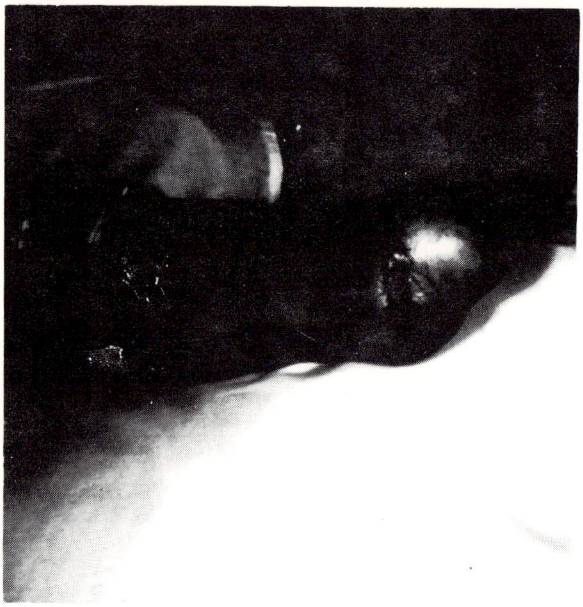

FIGURE 4-17

Amputation of foot through the talus and calcaneous. (Courtesy of Leon Cohen, D.P.M., Carlsbad, N.M.)

Metastasis

The longer the duration of the ulcer of squamous cell carcinoma, the greater the chance of metastasis to regional lymph nodes. Taylor, et al, (1941) believe metastasis of squamous carcinoma is rare even when associated with chronic osteomyelitis.[141] Whereas metastasis to regional nodes is unusual, it is still one of the chief therapeutic problems.[23] Frieden (1949) thinks one should assume that regional nodes may be involved eventually and dissection should be carried out.[47] Metastatic lesions may appear in the viscera, especially the liver, lungs and skin.[80] DeBell and Stevenson (1936) dissected all palpable nodes and 50.2% were found to be involved with metastasis.[40] Two centimeters is generally considered a "critical" size for squamous cell carcinoma in most areas of the body; lesions larger than this metastasize frequently, those smaller only occasionally.[53]

Squamous carcinoma arising in pre-existing skin lesions have a propensity for greater metastasis then those arising in sun-damaged skin.[54] Those arising in sun-exposed skin have a propensity to metastasize at about 0.5%.[96]

Distribution and Occurrence on the Foot

In a study of 511 skin tumors of the foot, Levene (1958) found 68 squamous cell carcinomas. Thirty-one appeared on the sole. The site of predilection was the metatarsal and heel area.[90] The foot is not generally a favored site for the occurrence of squamous cell carcinoma, although it is found more often than basal cell carcinoma. The obvious reason is because the foot is not exposed to prolonged sunlight. However, the foot and lower extremity are prone to chronic irritation, particularly in the heel and metatarsal area. The incidence of these lesions in areas of constant trauma must be kept in mind since the rate of metastasis is greater in these areas. Old burn scars, chronic osteomyelitis and stasis ulcer must be scrutinized for developing neoplasms.

Glass, et al, (1964) found the foot involved in 8 of 13 observed cases of the lower extremity even though the foot represents only 13% of the surface area of the lower extremity. The 8 tumors developed primarily from the normal skin of the foot. That is, no antecedent benign condition was recognized. The author concluded that primary carcinomas of the lower extremity occur most likely in the foot. "The high incidence of metastasis observed with these lesions can in part be correlated with the long duration of symptoms and large size obtained before they are biopsied and treated definitively."[53]

A study by Browne, et al, (1953) found 55 out of 511 squamous cell carcinoma in the foot. This represented 32.9% of the 614 lesions involving the lower extremity. Out of a total of 511 cases, 364 (71.7%) began with a precancerous lesion of some type.[22]

Treatment

The clinician experienced with either radiation, chemotherapy or surgery should be able to choose what method of treatment he prefers. This will depend on each individual case, with due regard to patients age and situation and the expertise of the therapist. Depth of lesion and histologic details are important considerations in treatment selection.

From a review of previous cure rates in 14,114 skin carcinomas, the great majority of epitheliomas can be cured with any of the standard methods.[37] Most surgeons prefer cold-knife surgery. Wide local excision is essential. Amputation, if osseous invasion occurs is often necessary.[54]

Treatment by electrodessication and currettage is another excellent therapy for the primary lesion uncomplicated by a previous, benign lesion. Tumors of approximately two cm or less are amenable to this treatment.[67] The merits are rapidity of treatment, no need for hospitalization, time saved, and good cosmetic results.

Since the prognosis of squamous cell carcinoma of the extremities is generally favorable due to its slow course and late metastatic rate, dissection of primary nodes following surgical excision is not universally accepted except if the squamous carcinoma occurs in the lower extremity where metastatic rate is high. Some surgeons dissect lymph nodes if palpable, or if there is any evidence of recurrence.[22,76] The significance of groin metastasis in squamous carcinoma of the lower extremity cannot be overemphasized.[54] In 60% of patients who had a groin dissection for clinical or histologic positive nodes, the cancer was permanently controlled.[54]

One must guard against the tendency to manage malignant ulcers as benign ones. Adequate sections on surgical excision should be requested of the pathologist by every surgeon excising skin cancers.[54] The report of inadequate wide excision warrants immediate wide re-excision or definite radiotherapy in an attempt to reduce the 80% recurrence rate and 25% mortality associated with these lesions. The attempt should be particularly aggressive in lesions greater than two cm in diameter. If every squamous cell carcinoma was removed with a one cm gross margin before the primary neoplasm exceeded a dimension of two cm, many unfortunate recurrences would be prevented. Cosmetic reconstruction should be delayed until control of the primary cancer has been ascertained.

Whenever possible, especially in large medical centers, the best results are seen by the dermatologist or surgical oncologist. They have more treatment methods at their command for skin lesions than any other medical specialist.

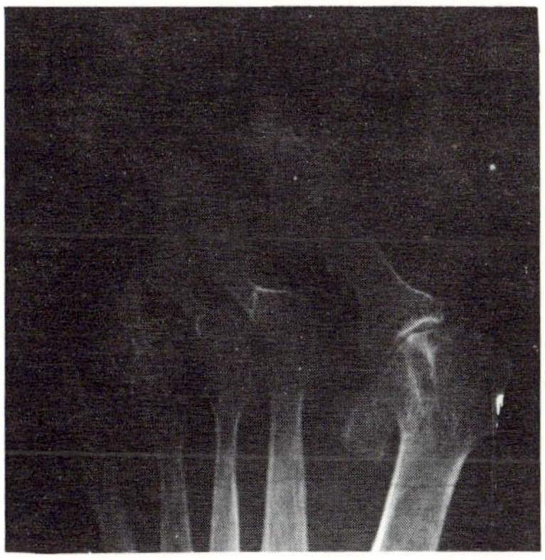

FIGURE 4-18

Squamous cell carcinoma involving hallux toe. Previous history of paronychia for over two years. Bone Involvement

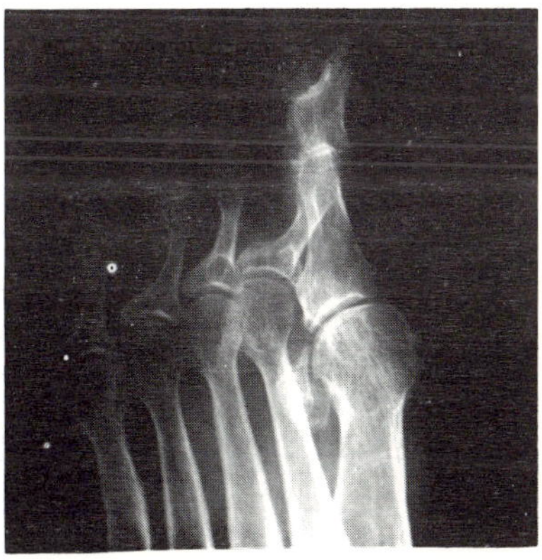

FIGURE 4-19

Secondary bone infiltration of squamous cell and osteomyelitis completely involving distal phalanx.

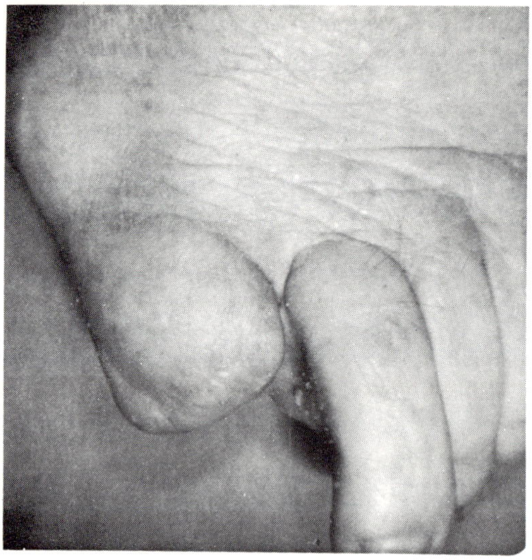

FIGURE 4-20

Amputation of distal phalanx and portion of proximal phalanx. Photo is 5 weeks post operative.

Prognosis

Prognosis is generally favorable depending on site. The disease usually runs a slow course and tends to metastasize late, but some of the most anaplastic and widely disseminating squamous cell carcinoma of the skin occur in old burn scars. No one need to die of squamous cell carcinoma of the skin.

Bowen's Disease (Intra-Epidermal Squamous Cell Carcinoma, Squamous Cell Carcinoma In Situ)

INTRODUCTION

Bowen's Disease (BD) is an eponymic designation for an intra-epidermal malignant neoplasm that is fairly characteristic clinically and highly characteristic histologically. Bowen described the condition in 1912, and since then many cases have been seen with similar clinical and histological features affecting many parts of the body.

It is characterized by a persistent, progressive, nonelevated, red, scaly or crusted plaque of the surface epidermis. It is relatively uncommon on the foot, but occurs on exposed and uncovered areas and may localize at sites of repeated trauma.

Etiology

1. Sunlight
2. Trivalent Arsenic Compounds[135, 137] — This is an important predisposing cause of BD. Graham et al present data that strongly suggests arsenic as one of the causes of BD, with an association with internal cancer.[59]

Sources of Arsenic — In the United Kingdom the majority of the cases with a history of arsenic exposure have been treated for psoriasis with Fowler's solution (potassium arsenic). In the U.S. it is the basis for Gay's solution, a treatment for asthma.[60] Agricultural workers may be exposed to arsenic salts used as fungicide weed-killer, sheep-dip or pesticide. Frequently the precautions taken against accidental ingestion or inhalation are inadequate. It has been the experience of many that very few patients admit exposure to arsenic on direct questioning.[125] On detailed and precise occupational and past medical history, a greater percentage provide suggestive evidence of exposure. In more than half the patients, however, the history does not suggest the cause. Yeh et al stated that in a limited area on the southwest coast of Taiwan, with a population of about 100,000, artesian wells are a source of drinking water for more than 45 years now.[151] Among the inhabitants of this area a remarkable percentage of chronic arsenic ingestion has manifested as hyperpigmentation, keratosis, and cancer. Of 238 arsenical skin cancers histologically studied, 46 were epidermoid carcinomas, 36 were basal cell carcinomas, 139 were intra-epidermal carcinomas (18 keratoses and 121 classic Bowen's lesions and varients) and 17 were combined forms.

Relationship to Internal Cancer

In 1959 Graham and Helwig reported a study of the relationship between BD and visceral cancer.[59] In their study of 35 patients with BD who came to autopsy or who died after surgical pathological examination of internal organs, 28 (80%) were observed to have one or more primary internal cancers of the skin, with metastases at an interval averaging 8.5 years after the appearance of Bowen's disease. Of those patients still living, 23 of more than 100 were found to have associated internal malignant disease. The disease involved predominately older age groups. Average duration from onset of BD to removal was 7.8 years. They appeared as lenticular, polycyclic, erythematous, pigmented, crusty, scaly, keratotic, nodular and ulcerated plaques and were sharply demarcated from the surrounding tissue. Correct clinical diagnosis was usually some variety of carcinoma.

In 1961, Peterka et al reported follow-up on 53 patients in whom BD was diagnosed during 1941-55.[120] Their findings indicated that the incidence of internal cancer is significantly increased in patients with BD occuring on a covered area of the body. The lack of correlation between the existence of internal cancer and BD on exposed surfaces may be due to the difficulty in clearly establishing a diagnosis of BD in exposed areas.

Goldman reported two cases of BD and carcinoma of the lung, one of which had arsenicism. Both patients had developed unusual clinical courses for lung carcinoma. The illness was fatal in both. The association between BD and lung carcinoma needs reemphasizing. One patient, age 47, was taking Fowler's solution for treatment of asthma since 12 years of age. She had palmoplantar hyperkeratosis as an associated finding. Arsenic can cause mottled brown-grayish hyperpigmentation and/or keratosis of the palms and soles.

The evidence favoring an association of BD and internal malignancy is increasing. All persons with BD should therefore, have repeated, thorough examinations for internal cancer, particularly in those cases where the cutaneous involvement appeared on the unexposed areas. Such examinations may be expected to contribute to earlier recognition of asymptomatic internal cancer.

Histologic Appearance

Bowen's disease is characterized histologically by atypical squamous cell proliferation throughout the thickness of the epidermis (squamous cell carcinoma in situ).[67] Variable acanthosis with increased length and thickness of the interpapillary ridges with retention of a distinct dermal-epidermal junction showing abnormal mitotic proliferation and mal-development of epidermal cells in the form of variation in size and shape are seen. If cells become invasive, they are almost always squamous cell in type. Invasion into the dermis is not usual, the basal cell remaining intact and metastatic spread is unlikely. When there is dermal invasion, a true squamous cell carcinoma results which affects both the diagnosis and prognosis. If dermal invasion is a possibility, serial tissue section is advisable.[60]

Clinical Picture

Bowen's disease, as a rule, manifests as a single, patchy lesion arising spontaneously. The lesion may occur anywhere on the skin surface or mucous membrane. The initial change is a small dull-brownish to red patch or scaly area of sharp irregular outline with little or no infiltration. Secondary crusting and oozing may appear beneath the crust. It is usually asymptomatic and gradually enlarges in a somewhat irregular fashion peripherally with no signs of central ulceration. The scale is white or yellowish, detached without much trouble to give a moist, reddened, and at times granular surface without producing bleeding. The margin is usually sharp and the lesion slightly raised. Ulceration is usually a sign of invasion into the dermis; it may be delayed for many years after the appearance of the intra-epidermal change.[125] Persistent superficial ulceration may be an early indication of BD of the palmar or plantar skin without invasion.

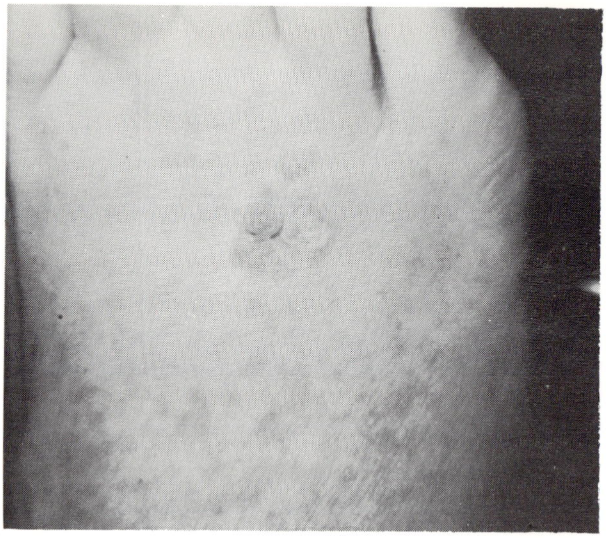

FIGURE 4-21

Bowen's Disease: GDorsal aspect of foot revealing hyperkeratotic scale. Recurrent lesion from previous therapy.

Incidence on the Pedal Extremity

Bowen's disease of the foot is extremely rare. Perhaps not often reported or undiagnosed would be more accurate. The number of reported cases in the literature are not readily available; much searching was required to report on even the following cases.

Chaudheim and Panja reported a case in a 32 year old female with solid elevations and firmly adherent crusts on the soles dorsum of right foot, left thigh and forearm.[26] The lesions on the sole were ulcerated, showing clear-cut margins. Histopathologic evidence of Bowen's disease was present. This case was reported from Calcutta where available records do not show any incidence of Bowen's disease in India. Other unusual features are the multiple painful lesions and involvement of the soles.

Another case of Bowen's disease of the foot was reported in a 58-year old female.[74] The specific foot area was not given. Length of treatment was one month before desired results were obtained. The follow-up had been for seven months.

Nail bed epithelium involvement is very rare.[34] A review of the past 20 years of world literature of Bowen's disease of the nail bed revealed only a few reported cases. One case involved the hallux nail.[34] It occurred in a 67 year old female with an 8 mm ulcer with heaped up edges present for five years. Destruction of the overlying nail plate was evident. The typical case of a bowenoid lesion on non-pedal skin is characterized by well-defined erythematous plaques with a super-imposed yellowish crust. Bowen's disease of the nail bed manifests differently. The important clinical feature is *nail plate absence in a specific area with irregular thickening or ulceration of the bed.* Nail matrix involvement may be present.

Recently, Rubin reported an additional case of nail bed involvement.[127] A 77 year old male presented with a granular, verrucose appearing lesion, gray white in color, of the third toenail. The lesion was present for three years and treated unsuccessfully previously. After histologic examination, the toe was amputated at the distal phalanx.

Genoveses (1974) reported an unusual location of Bowen's disease involving the fourth interspace.[50] A 55 year old male, with a possible previous history of arsenic exposure, presented with what clinically was a heloma molle. The lesion was large, thickened, elevated, white and wrinkled in appearance as a result of maceration. Fissuring of the lesion and sulcus of the fifth toe was present. Treatment for fungal infection, debridement and pads to separate the toes were tried. After several months, the area became ulcerated and inflamed. Excision and grafting of the toe interspace was performed and Bowen's disease was reported.

Differential Diagnosis

1. Lichen simplex-papular, uncomplicated eruption.
2. Psoriasis and other eczematous dermatosis - BD resembles an eczematous or psoriasiform lesion, but does not respond to the treatment of eczema or psoriasis. If the diagnosis is uncertain, the lack of improvement with steroid therapy is suggestive of BD.
3. Superficial basal cell carcinoma - This tumor can produce a very similar appearance, but can usually be differentiated by the finely elevated thread-like margin. BD and superficial basal cell carcinoma can be seen simultaneously in the same patient.
4. Solar keratosis (flat type - present as smaller lesions than

BD with an atypical basal cell layer. Their presence on the foot is extremely rare, if at all.

5. Arsenical keratosis - same as for solar keratosis.
6. Nail bed involvement - includes:[34]
   a. verruca
   b. onychomycosis
   c. granuloma pyogenicum
   d. glomus tumor
   e. subungual exostosis
   f. keratoacanthoma
   g. squamous cell carcinoma
   h. amelanotic melanoma

Treatment

In general, one should use the technique which he finds most suitable, if the end result is acceptable by both the therapist and the patient.

Destruction of the epidermis by adequate freezing, cauterization or diathermy coagulation is often effective. Radiotherapy has to be in full tumor doses and is likely to cause obvious scarring and possible radionecrosis in large lesions. Adequate doses of grenz ray therapy can also be employed successfully.

Local cytotoxic agents such as 5-flourouracil can be applied with good results.[48]

Recurrences are not infrequent and may come from extension of the cancer in situ around appendage ducts which were not affected by the original treatment.

Surgical excision is a good treatment if the lesion is not too large.[59] It is indicated, in general, in any superficial growth that may be removed by simple excision, as an office procedure, provided the skin edges can be approximated after excision. Obviously the size of the lesion that can be excised will vary with location and patient's age. Whenever a suspected BD is small enough, excisional surgery should be complete for purpose of treatment and biopsy.[44] Surgical curettement may also be employed.

Honeycott and Jansen treated 52 patients with BD (only one case on the foot) by electrodessication and curettage (ED&C) with only one recurrence. Follow-up studies were done for a minimum of four years. Most of the lesions were less than 2 cm and the one recurrence was of greater than 2 cm. The authors state that most older textbooks of dermatology advocate surgery as the recommended treatment. The new texts suggest ED&C as effective therapy, but a preliminary biopsy is essential. The authors believe ED&C is best for the treatment of BD from the standpoint of cure, cosmetic result and simplicity. Lesions greater than 2 cm in size would require grafting if surgically excised, and this would require more technical time, expense, and a less acceptable cosmetic result.

BIBLIOGRAPHY

1. Ackerman, L. V. and del Regato, J. A.: *Cancer,* Ed. 3, C. V. Mosby, Co. St. Louis, p. 167-210.
2. Allen, A. C. and Spritz, S.: Malignant melanoma, a clinicopathological analysis of criteria for diagnosis and prognosis. *Cancer,* **6**:1, 1953.
3. Alrich, E. M.: Isolation perfusion. *Amer. J. of Surg.,* **21**:583, 1971.
4. Becker, S. W.: Pigmented epitheliomas. *Arch. Derm. Syph.,* **27**:981, 1933.
5. Becker, S. W.: Benign epidermal neoplasma. *Arch. Derm. Syph.,* **26**:838, 1932.
6. Becker, W.: Pitfalls in the diagnosis and treatment of melanoma. *Arch. Derm. Syph.,* **69**:11, 1954.
7. Behrman, H. T., Lebow, T. A., and Rozen, J. H.: *Common Skin Diseases – Diagnosis and Treatment,* 2nd ed. Groune and Strotton, Inc., N.Y., 1971, Section III, p. 149-159.
8. Belisario, J.: Malignant melanoblastomas, some usual and unusual aspects and vagaries. *Aust. J. Derm.,* **8**:224, 1966.
9. Berger, R. A., Auerbach, R., and Orentreich, N.: Basal cell epithelioma of the sole, *Arch. Derm.,* **94**:317-319, 1966.
10. Bick, Em. M.: Primary carcinomas of the extremities. *Ann. Surg.,* **103**:410, 1932.
11. Binkley, G. W. and Rauschkalb, R. R.: Basal cell epithelioma metastasizing to lymph nodes. *Arch. Derm.,* **86**:332, 1962.
12. Block, G. E. and Hartwell, S. W.: Malignant melanoma: A study of 217 cases. *Ann. Surg.,* **154**:74, 1961.
13. Blum, H. F.: Sunlight as an environmental factor in cancer of the skin. *Milit. Med.,* **117**:202, 1955.
14. Bodenham, D. C.: Malignant melanoma — some observations on the nature of the disease and their implications. *Med. J. Aust.,* **58**:271, 1971.
15. Booner, R. J.: Recognition and treatment of melanoma. *Surg. Clinics of N. Amer.,* **49**(2):389, 1969.
16. Booner, R. J. and Pack, G. T.: Malignant melanoma of the feet and hands. *Surg.,* **42**(6):1084, 1957.
17. Bornstein, B.: Subungual melanoma, a case report., *JAPA,* **49**(12):528, 1959.
18. Bowen, J. T.: Precancerous dermatoses: a study of two cases of chronic atypical epithelial proliferation. *J. Cut. Dis.,* **30**:241-255, 1912.
19. Bower, R. F., and Young, J. M.: Carcinoma arising in scars, osteomyelitis and fistulas. *Arch. Surg.,* **80**:564, 1960.

20. Broders, A. C.: Squamous cell epithelioma of the skin: A study of 256 cases. *Ann. Surg.,* **73**:141, 1921.
21. Broders, A. C.: Practical points of the malignant grading of carcinoma. *N.Y.J. Med.,* **32**:667, 1932.
22. Browne, H. J., Coventry, M. B., and McDonald, J. R.: Squamous carcinoma of the extremities. *Staff Meet. of the Mayo Clinic,* **28**:590, 1953.
23. Campanelli, M.: Juvenile melanoma — a case report. *JAPA,* **56**(10):461, 1966.
24. Charache, H.: Squamous cell carcinoma of the extremities. *Surg. Gynec. & Obst.,* **68**:1002, 1939.
25. Charalambidis, P. H. and Patterson, W. B.: A clinical study of 250 patients with malignant melanoma. *Surg. Gynec. and Obstet.,* **115**:333, 1962.
26. Chaudhuri, S. H. and Panja, G.: Bowen's disease: A case report. *Brit. J. Derm.,* **71**:117, 1959.
27. Cholnoky, T.: Malignant melanoma — 117 cases. *Ann. Surg.,* **113**:392, 141.
28. Clark, W. and Mihm, M.: Lentigo maligna and lentigo-maligna melanoma. *Amer. J. Path.,* **55**:39, 1969.
29. Clark, W. and Mihm, M.: Histogenesis and biologic behavior of primary human malignant melanoma of the skin. *Cancer Res.,* **29**:705, 1969.
30. Clarke, H. M.: Primary carcinoma of the extremity. *Surg. Gynec. Obst.,* **79**:669, 1944.
31. Conley, J.: Irradiation as an etiologic factor in the development of melanoma. *Arch. Otolaryngol.,* **92**:627, 1970.
32. Conrad, F. G.: Treatment of malignant melanoma. *Arch. Surg.,* **104**:587, 1972.
33. Cook, R. T.: Malignant melanoma of the skin and mucous membrane. *J. Kansas Med. Soc.,* **64**:440, 1963.
34. Coskey, R. J., Mehregan, A., and Fosnough, R.: Bowen's disease of the nail *Bed. Arch. Derm.,* **106**:79, 1972.
35. Cowdell, R. H.: Cutaneous hematoma simulating melanoma. *Brit. J. Surg.,* **44**:545, 1957.
36. Creech, Krementz, Ryan and Winblad: Chemotherapy of cancer: Regional perfusion utilizing an extracorporeal circuit. *Ann. Surg.,* **148**:616, 1958.
37. Crissey, J. T.: Curettage and electrodesiccation as a method of treatment for epitheliomas of the skin. *J. Surg. Oncol.,* **3**:287, 1971.
38. Daj Gupta, T. and Brasfield, R.: Subungual melanoma — 25 year review of cases. *Ann. Surg.,* **116**:545, 1965.
39. Daland, E. M.: Malignant melanoma. *New Eng. J. Med.,* **260**:453, 1959.
40. DeBell, P. J., and Stevenson, T. D.: Squamous cell epithelioma of the extremities. *Surg. Gynec. & Obst.,* **63**:222, 1936.
41. Decker, A. M. and Chamness, J. T.: Melanocarcinoma of the plantar surface of the foot. *Surg.* **29**:731, 1951.
42. Downing, J. G.: Cancer of the skin and occupational trauma. *JAMA,* **148**:245, 1952.
43. Epstein, E.: Biopsy and prognosis of malignant melanoma. *JAMA,* **208**:1396, May, 1969.
44. Epstein, E.: *Skin Surgery,* 3rd ed. C. C. Thomas Publishers, Springfield, 1970.
45. Fortner, J. G., Booner, R. J., and Pack, G. T.: Results of groin dissection for malignant melanoma in 220 patients. *Surg.,* **55**:485, 1964.
46. Foulds, L.: The histological analysis of tumors. *Am. J. Cancer,* **39**:1, 1940.

47. Frieden, J. H.: The regional lymph node dissection in cancer of the extremities. *Surg. Gynec. & Obst.,* **89**:591, 1949.
48. Fulton, J. E., Carter, D. M., and Hurley, H. J.: Treatment of Bowen's disease with topical 5-fluorurocil under occlusion. *Arch. Derm.* **97**:178-180, 1968.
49. Galinski, A.: Noles and malignant melanoma. *JAPA,* **63**:35, 1973.
50. Genoveses, V. H.: Heloma molle — Bowen's Disease. *JAPA,* **64**:108, 1974.
51. Gerstein, W.: Transplantation of basal cell epithelioma to the rabbit. Arch. Derm., **88**:834, 1963.
52. Ghadially, F. N.: Pathology: Trauma and melanoma production. *Nature* (London), **21**:1199, 1966.
53. Glass, R. L., Spratt, J. S., and Perez-Mesa, C.: Epidermoid carcinoma of the lower extremities. *Arch. Surg.,* **89**:955, 1964.
54. Glass, R. L., Spratt, J. S., and Perez-Mesa, C.: Fate of inadequately excised epidermoid carcinomas of the skin. *Surg. Gynec. & Obst.,* **122**:245, 1966.
55. Gold, R.: Basal cell carcinoma. *JAPA,* **57**:128-129, March, 1967.
56. Goldmon, A. L.: Lung cancer in Bowen's Disease. *Am. Rev. Respir. Disease,* **108**:1205-1207, 1973.
57. Goldner, R.: Carcinoma developing in lupus erythematosis scar, *S. Med. Journ.,* **62**:733, 1969.
58. Goldsmith, N. S., Shah, J. P., and Kim, D.: Malignant melanoma: Current concepts of lymph node dissection. *Cancer,* **22**:216, 1972.
59. Graham, J. H. and Helwig, E. B.: Bowen's Disease and its relationship to systemic cancer. *Arch. Derm.,* **80**:133-159, 1959.
60. Graham, J. H., Mazzunt, G. R., and Helwig, E. B.: Chemistry of Bowen's Disease: its relationship to arsenic. *J. invest. Derm.,* **37**:317-330, 1961.
61. Gumpert, S., and Meyer, H.: Treatment of 126 cases of malignant melanoma, long term results. *Ann. Surg.,* **150**:989, 1959.
62. Hall, J. R., Phillips, C. and White, R. P.: Melanoma — a study of 222 cases. *Surg. Gynec. and Obst.,* **95**:184, 1952.
63. Handley, W. S.: Hunterian lectures on the pathology of melanotic growths in relation to the operative treatment. *Lancet,* **1**:996, 1907.
64. Harnett, W. L.: *A Survey of Cancer in London.* Brit. Empire Cancer Campaign. London, 1952.
65. Harter, J. G. and Novitch, A. M.: An evaluation of Gay's solution in the treatment of asthma. *J. Allergy,* **40**:327-336, 1967.
66. Heller, A. G.: A prophylactic surgical procedure. *JAPA,* **48**:258, 1958.
67. Honeycott, W. M. and Jansen, T. C.: Treatment of squamous cell carcinoma of the Skin. *Arch. Derm.,* **108**:670, 1973.
68. Hueston, J. T.: Integumentectomy for malignant melanoma of the limbs. *Aust. N.Z. J. Surgery,* **40**(2):114, 1970.
69. Hunter, G. A., and Hellier, F. F.: Tumors of palm and sole resembling basal cell epithelioma. *Brit. J. Derm.,* **72**:285-287, 1960.
70. Hutchinson, J.: On senile moles and senile freckles and on their relationship to the cancerous process. *Arch. Surg.,* **2**:218, 1890.
71. Hyman, A. B. and Michaelides, P.: Basal cell epithelioma of the sole. *Arch. Derm.,* **87**:481-485, 1963.
72. Jackson, R.: Colloquium on cutaneous malignant melanoma. *Comad. Med. Assoc. Journ.,* **99**:1, 1968.
73. Jackson, R.: Lentigo maligna and malignant melanoma. *Comad. Med. Assoc. Journ.,* **95**:846, 1966.

74. Jansen, C. T., Dillaha, C. J., and Honeycott, W. M.: Bowenoid conditions of the skin. *Southern Med. J.*, **60**:185, 1967.
75. Jones, R. F. and Dickinson, W. E.: Total integumentectomy of the leg for multiple "in-transit" metastases of melanoma. *Am. J. Surg.*, **123**:588, 1972.
76. Kimbrough, R. F., Coventry, M. B., and McDonald, J. R.: Squamous Carcinoma of the Extremity. *S. Clin. North Amer.*, **31**:1179, 1951.
77. Kirsch, N.: Malignant melanoma in a tattoo. *Int. J. Derm.*, **11**:16, 1972.
78. Kloppl C. T.: Fractionated intra-arterial cancer chemotherapy with methyl bis Amine HC1. *Ann. Surg.*, **B2**:811, 1950.
79. Knutson, C. O., et al: Melanoma. *Curr. Probl. Surg.*, Dec., 1971.
80. Kulchar, C. V.: Benign and malignant tumors of the foot. *JAMA*, **124**:761, 1944.
81. Lancaster, H. O. and Nelson, J.: Sunlight as a cause of melanoma: A clinical survey. *Med. J. Aust.*, **44**:452, 1957.
82. Langdon: Melanosarcoma of the sole of the foot. *Am. J. Surg.*, **IV**:170, 1894.
83. Lea, A. J.: Malignant melanoma of the skin: The relationship to trauma. *Ann. Roy. Coll. Surg. Eng.*, **37**:169, 1965.
84. Leading Article: Malignant melanoma. *Brit. Med. J.*, **2**:129, 1967.
85. Leading Article: The junctional nevus. *Cancer Bull.* (Tex.), **9**:22, 1957.
86. Lee, J. and Merrill, J. M.: Sunlight and the etiology of malignant melanoma: A synthesis. *Med. J. Aust.*, **2**:846, 1970.
87. Lee, J. and Merrill, J. M.: Sunlight and melanoma. *Lancet*, **2**:550, 1971.
88. Lehman, et al: Clinical study of 49 patients with malignant melanoma. *Cancer*, **19**:611, 1966.
89. Levene, A.: Etiology of vitiligo —*Lancet*, **1**:263, 1972.
90. Levene, M.: Distribution of skin tumors of the sole of the foot. *Brit. Med. J.*, **19**:1519, 1958.
91. Lever, W. F.: *Histopathology of the Skin.* 4th ed. J. B. Lippincott, Co., Phila. 1967.
92. Lever, W. F.: Pathogenesis of benign tumors of cutaneous appendages and of basal cell epithelioma. *Arch. Derm. Sypth.*, **57**:679, 1948.
93. Levit, F.: Malignant melanoma — A brief review of the pertinent literature. *Q. Bull. Northwest U. Med. School*, **32**:140, 1958.
94. Lewis, H. M., Stensaas, C. O., and Okun, M. R.: Basal cell epithelioma of the sole, *Arch. Derm.*, **91**:622-623, 1965.
95. Lewis, M. G.: Malignant melanoma in uganda. *Brit. J. Cancer.*, **21**:483, 1967.
96. Lund, H. Z.: How often does Squamous Cell Carcinoma of the skin metastasize. *Arch. Derm.*, **92**:635, 1965.
97. Lund, R. H. and Ihnen: Malignant melanoma: Clinical and pathologic analysis of 93 cases. *Surgery*, **38**:652, 1955.
98. McCarthy, J. G.: The role of groin dissection in the management of patients with melanoma of the lower extremity. *Rev. of Surgery*, **28**:374, 1971.
99. McLeod, R., et al: Retrospective survey of patients with malignant melanoma. *Surg. Gynec. and Obst.*, **126**:99, 1968.
100. McNeer and DasGupta: Malignant melanoma. *Surg. Clin. N. Amer.*, **49**:389, 1969.
101. McPeak, C. J., McNeer, G. P., Whiteley, H. W., and Booner, R. J.: Amputation for melanoma of the extremity. *Surgery*, **54**:426, 1963.
102. Mehnert, J. and Heard, J. L.: Staging of malignant melanoma by depth or invasion. *Am. J. Surg.*, **110**:168, 1965.

103. Meyer, H. W. and Gumport, S. L.: Malignant melanoma appraisal of the disease and analysis of 105 cases. *Ann. Surg.,* **138**:643, 1953.
104. Midkiff, L. C.: Malignant melanoma, a case history. *J. Nat. Assoc. of Chiropodists,* **47**(12):613, 1957.
105. Milton, G. W. and Brown, M. M.: Malignant melanoma — two problems. *Aust. J. Derm.,* **9**:157, 1967.
106. Montgomery, H.: In discussion of Goldman, H. J.: Multiple benign cystic epithelioma. *JAMA,* **115**:2253, 1940.
107. Moore, C.: *Synopsis of Clinical Cancer,* 2nd ed., C. V. Mosby, Co., St. Louis 1970, ch. 1-4.
108. Morris, G. C. and Horn, R. C.: Malignant melanoma in the negro. *Surgery,* **29**:223, 1951.
109. Mundth, E. D., Guralanick, E. A., and Raker, J. W.: Malignant melanoma: A clinical study of 427 cases. *Ann. Surg.,* **162**:15, 1965.
110. Okun, M. R.: Malignant melanoma arising from an intradermal nevus. *Arch. Derm.* (Chicago), **92**:69, 1965.
111. Okun, M. R. and Ansell, H. R.: Eccrine poroma. *Arch. Derm.,* **88**:561-566, 1963.
112. Olsen, G.: Removal of fascia — cause of more frequent metastases of malignant melanoma of the skin to regional lymph nodes? *Cancer,* **17**:1159, 1964.
113. Olsen, G.: Malignant melanoma of the skin. *Danish Med. Bull.,* **KL**:229, 1967.
114. Pack, et al: Principle of excision and dissection in continuity for primary and metastatic melanoma of the skin. *Surgery,* **17**:849, 1945.
115. Pack, G. T. and Adair, F. E.: Subungual melanoma. *Surgery,* **5**:47, 1939.
116. Pack, G. T., Gerber, D. M., and Scharnagel, I.: End results of treatment of malignant melanoma, a report of 1190 cases. *Ann. Surg.,* **136**:905, 1952.
117. Pack, G. T., Gerber, D. M., and Scharnagel, I.: Treatment of malignant melanoma — report of 862 cases. *Calif. Med.,* **66**:283, 1947.
118. Pascher, F. and Sims, C. F.: Basal cell epitheliomas of the sole. *Arch. Derm.,* **69**:475-481, 1954.
119. Perzik, S. L. and Barim, R. K.: Individualization in the management of melanomas: A review of 164 consecutive cases. *Am. Surgeon,* **35**:177, 1969.
120. Peterka, E. S., Lynch, F. W., Goltz, R. W.: Association between Bowen's Disease and internal cancer. *Arch. Derm.,* **84**:623-629, 1961.
121. Pinkus, H.: Premaligant fibroepithelial tumors of the skin. *A.M.A. Arch. Derm. Syph.,* **67**:598, 1953.
122. Pinkus, H., Rogin, J. R., and Goldman, P.: Eccrine poroma, *Arch. Derm.,* **74**:511, 1956.
123. Potter, J.: Management of nevi and melanomas. *Amer. Surg.,* **36**:261, 1970.
124. Pringle, J. H.: A method of operation in cases of melanotic tumors of the skin. *Edinburgh Med. J.,* **23**:496, 1908.
125. Rook, A., Wilkinson, D. S., Ebling, F. J. G.: *Textbook of Dermatology,* Vol. 2, 2nd ed. Blackwell Scientific Publications, London, 1972, p. 1962-1964.
126. Rosenberg, H.: Seborrheic keratosis or basal cell carcinoma. *JAPA,* **54**:478-480, 1964.
127. Rubin, L.: Intraepidermal squamous cell carcinoma (Bowen's Disease) of the nail bed. *JAPA,* **63**:195, 1973.
128. Sachs, W. and Garbe, W.: Primary basal cell epitheliomas of the extremities. *Arch. Derm. and Syph.,* **36**:273,1937.

129. Sauer, G. C.: *Manual of Skin Diseases,* 2nd ed. J. B. Lippincott Co., Phila., 1959.

130. Schoch, E. P.: Familial malignant melanoma. *Arch. Derm.* (Chicago), **88**:445, 1963.

131. Schreiner, B. F. and Wehr, W. H.: Primary malignant tumors of the foot. *Radiology,* **21**:513, 1933.

132. Schrek, R.: Cutaneous epithelioma: III, A statistical analysis with respect to site, sex and pre-existing scars. *Arch. Path.,* **31**:434-448, 1941.

133. Sears, F. W.: Vicevated malignant melanoma of the foot. *JAPA,* **62**(4):156, 1972.

134. Sedlin, E. D. and Fleming, J. L.: Epidermoid carcinoma in chronic osteomyelitic foci. *J. Bone & Joint Surg.,* **45A**:827, 1963.

135. Seiji, M. and Mizuno, F.: Electron microscopic study of Bowen's Disease. *Arch. Derm.,* **99**:3, 1969.

136. Shapiro, L. and Bodran, E.: Malignant melanoma in the form of pedunculated papsles. *Arch. Derm.,* **99**:49, 1969.

137. Sommers, S. C. and McManus, R. G.: Multiple arsenical cancer of skin and internal organs. *Cancer,* **6**:347-359, 1953.

138. Stegmaier, O. C.: Life cycle of the nevus. *Modern Med.,* **31**(13):79, 1963.

139. Stehlin, J. S.: Malignant melanoma: An appraisal. *Surg.,* **64**:1149, 1969.

140. Stehlin, J. S. and Clark, R. L.: Melanoma of the extremities. *Am. J. Surg.,* **110**:366, 1965.

141. Taylor, C. W., Nathanson, I. T., and Shaw, D. T.: Epidermoid carcinoma of the extremity with reference to lymph node involvement. *Ann. Surg.,* **113**:268, 1941.

142. Teloh, H. A. and Wheelock, M. C.: Histogensis of basal cell carcinoma. *Arch. Path.,* **48**:447, 1949.

143. Tompkins, V. N.: Cutaneous melanoma: vicevation as a prognostic sign. *Cancer,* **6**:1215, 1953.

144. Van Scott, E. J. and Reinertson, R. P.: The modulating influence of stromal environment on epithelial cells studied in human autotransplants. *J. Invest. Derm.,* **36**:109, 1961.

145. Waller, S. O.: Malignant melanoma presenting with bone metastasis and foot drop. *Med. J. Aust.,* **1**:271, 1971.

146. Watson, E. C.: Melanoma — a ten year retrospective survey in N. Zealand. *Aust. N. A. J. Surg.,* **33**:31, 1963.

147. Webster, J. P., et al: Surgical treatment of malignant melanoma of the skin. *Surg. Clin. N. Amer.,* **24**:319, 1944.

148. Weitzner, S.: Basal cell carcinoma of toeweb presenting as junctional nevus. *Southwest Med.,* **49**:175-177, October, 1968.

149. Williams, H. M.: Malignant melanoma. *Cancer,* **18**:151, 1968.

150. Williams, K. E. and Butcher, H. R.: Cutaneous carcinoma mistaken for stasis ulcer of the leg. *Amer. Surg.,* **27**:1, 1961.

151. Yeh, S., How, S. W., and Lin, C. S.: Arsenical cancer of skin: Histologic study with special reference to Bowen's Disease. *Cancer,* **21**:312-339, 1968.

152. Zelickson, A. S.: An electron microscope study of the basl cell epithelioma. *J. Invest. Derm.,* **39**:183, 1962.

153. Zugerman, I.: Basal cell epithelioma of the sole. *Arch. Derm.,* **76**:247-249, 1957.

SECTION V

TUMORS OF THE PEDAL SKIN AND RELATED CONNECTIVE TISSUE NEOPLASMS

Adnexal Tumors

Tumors of skin appendages are not uncommon lesions affecting the foot. They may arise from the eccrine glands, sebaceous glands, or the epidermis. These lesions are often misdiagnosed.

1. ECCRINE POROMA

Eccrine poroma usually presents as an asymptomatic, pink-to-red colored, pedunculated lesion which may be hyperkeratotic and occasionally bleeds. It is usually smaller than 1 cm and grows very slowly.[111,130] It may be sessile or slightly pedunculated.

Etiology

This benign skin tumor was first described in 1956, by Pinkus and associates, who believed it to be a neoplasm of the intra-

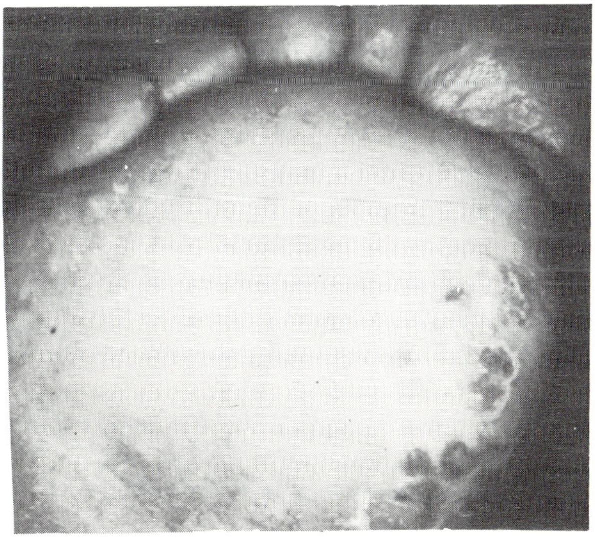

FIGURE 5-1

Multiple Eccrine Poromas: A rare condition revealing multiple eccrine poromas on the plantar surface of the foot and digits. (Courtesy of Ronald Goldner, M.D., Baltimore, Maryland.)

epidermal portion of the eccrine sweat duct, or acrosyringium.[103] This was confirmed by Sanderson and Ryan, who found high levels of glycogen and enzymes, characteristic of eccrine structures, in histochemical studies of the tumor.[115] Hyman and Brownstein reviewed 96 cases of eccrine poroma.[67] They feel that the tumor is not as rare as previously reported, since many of the lesions are misdiagnosed. Eccrine poroma is found usually in patients over age 40.[99] It is located in areas of glabrous skin which contain many eccrine glands, most often on the soles.[111] It is usually a solitary lesion but ulceration may occur under weight bearing areas of the foot. Goldner has reported a case of multiple eccrine poromas involving the foot.[50]

Histopathology

The tumor is primarily intra-epidermal, but may extend into the dermis in a pattern of pseudoepitheliomatous hyperplasis.[1] It is probably related to the dermal duct tumor reported by Winkelman.[58] It contains characteristic cuboidal cells in irregular, partially reticulated strands with intercellular bridging[19] It may show connections to an eccrine sweat duct.[111] Biopsy of the neoplasm is necessary for a proper diagnosis.

Differential Diagnosis

Differential diagnosis can be made both clinically and histologically and includes both benign and malignant lesions.[47,50,99,103] Previous failures in differential diagnosis probably account for the recent increase in reported cases of eccrine poroma. Benign lesions which resemble eccrine poroma are: verrucae plantaris, which is more hyperkeratotic than eccrine poroma; granuloma pyogenicum, which is more vascular; dermatofibroma, which is less vascular; epidermal nevus; hemangioma; and seborrheic keratosis. Callous lesions over weight bearing areas of the foot can easily be misdiagnosed and may include malignant lesions such as: basal cell carcinoma, which is rare on the sole; squamous cell carcinoma; Kaposi's sarcoma; and amelanotic melanoma.[148]

Prognosis

Adequate treatment insures a good prognosis. Recurrances after complete excision are rare. Complications, other than bleeding, are infrequent, and malignant transformation are very rare.

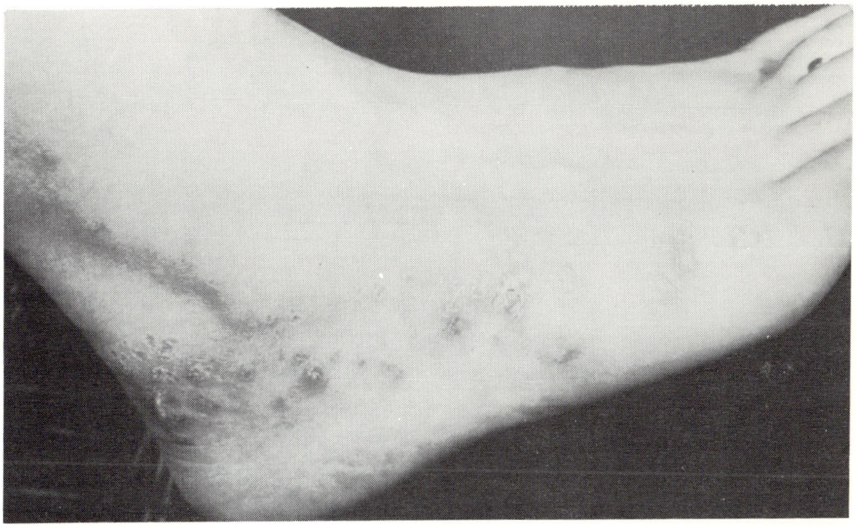

FIGURE 5-2

Linear Porokeratosis of Mibelli: Multiple lesions arranged in a linear fashion along border of the foot, usually asymptomatic, characterized by raised keratotic walls with a groove often filled with keratotic material (Courtesy of Ronald Goldner, M.D., Baltimore, Maryland.)

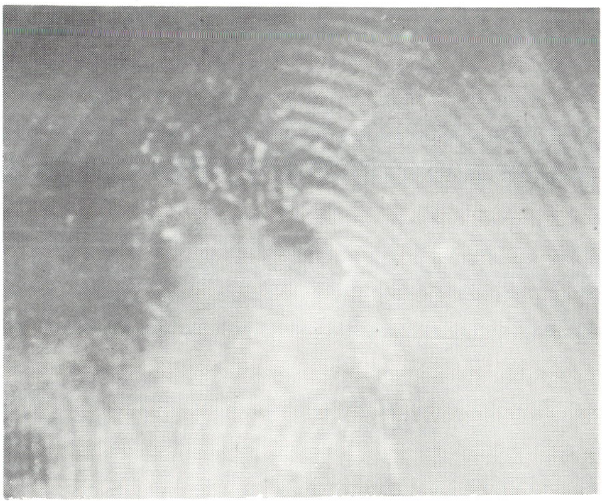

FIGURE 5-3

Eccrine Poroma: Early small ill-defined lesion on plantar surface of the foot. Treatment is by adequate excision of lesion and surrounding skin margins Plastic closures may be necessary to close defect.

Treatment

Most authors agree that surgical excision is the treatment of choice, provided an adequate margin or normal tissue is excised with the tumor.

2. POROKERATOSIS PLANTARIS DISCRETA

Porokeratosis plantaris discreta was first described by Taub and Steinberg in 1970 as a cyst which forms on the plantar surface of the foot as a consequence of eccrine sweat pore obstruction by callus tissue.[132] It was included in a discussion of benign skin neoplasms when Steinberg first described the lesion in 1951 as a "plugged duct cyst."[132] Histopathologic studies by Taub confirmed that the lesion was indeed a result of sweat pore obstruction which was present in 13.5% of 639 foot biopsies.[132] Previously this lesion has been identified as a "neurofibrous callus, intractable plantar keratosis (IPK), keratotic wart, burnt-out plantar wart, tyloma, or just plain callosity."[132]

Confusion often results because several other dermatological entities have names similar to porokeratosis plantaris discreta. Porokeratosis of Mibelli, first described in 1893, is a rare, familial condition thought to be a clonal disease of the eccrine epidermal cells.[104] The lesions are disc-shaped, widely disseminated, and can occur in any area of the body.[93] The disease is most common in males in the second and third decades.[116] Porokeratosis of Mantoux is a rare palmoplantar keratoderma of unknown etiology; crops of lesions on the palms and soles shed in a few weeks without complications.[59]

There is no apparent relationship between porokeratosis plantaris discreta and other tumors of the eccrine gland, ie.: eccrine nerves, eccrine hydrocystoma, syringoma, eccrine spiradenoma, eccrine poroma, and eccrine mixed tumor.[83]

Etiology

A pathomechanical imbalance in the foot can cause hyperkeratotic callous tissue to form over weight bearing areas such as the ball and heel. This thickened patch of tissue includes the pore of the eccrine gland; because the gland is under continued stimulation by the sympathetic nervous system, its fluid secretions

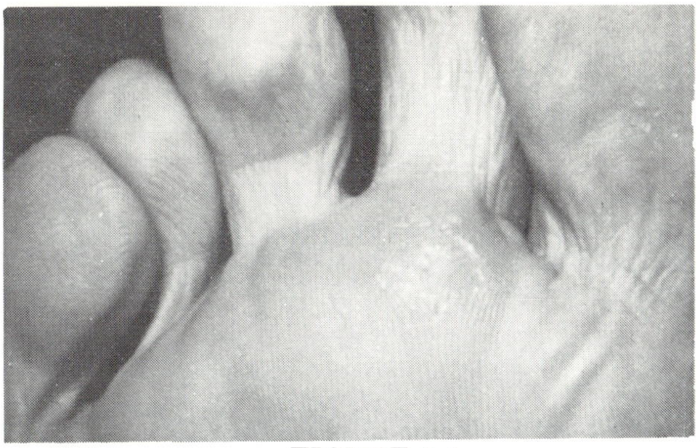

FIGURE 5-4

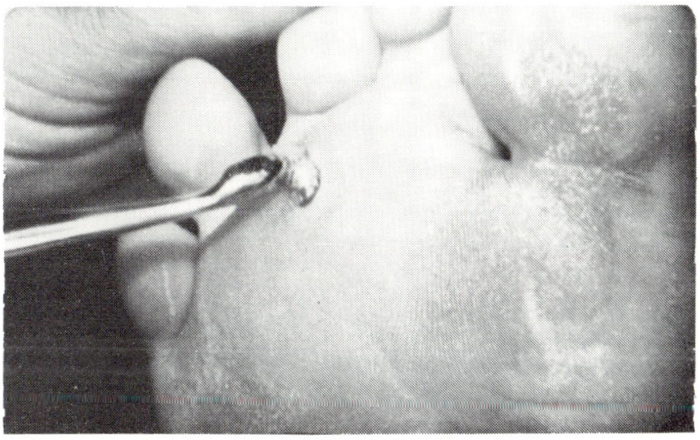

FIGURE 5-5

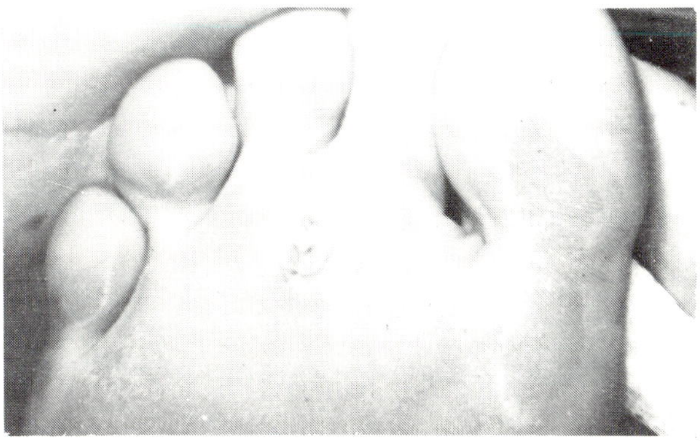

FIGURE 5-6

Porokeratosis Plantaris Discreta: This lesion is easily confused with both keratinous cysts and eccrine poroma. Treatment is by surgical excision.

"block up" into the deep portion of the duct causing dilitation and hypertrophy. Eventually the epidermal cells lining the sweat duct become keratinized, which results in a horny plug that causes pain by impingement on nerve endings in the dermis.[142]

Incidence

Porokeratosis plantaris discreta has only been described on the soles of the feet because this surface is exposed to considerable trauma and contains more eccrine glands than any area of the body.[28,94] The most common site is under the metatarsal heads. The cyst is usually found in adults of whom 75% are women.[132]

Clinical Considerations

After paring of the superficial callus, the lesion presents as a discrete, hyperkeratotic central plug of white-to-yellow material. It is found on weight-bearing areas, and is quite painful on both direct and lateral digital pressure.

Histopathology

Steinberg offers the best description of the lesion: cone-shaped and consisting of three epidermal components:

1. a superficial wide-base callus, 1 - 2 cm in diameter by 0.1 - 0.25 cm thick;
2. a tapering cornoid plug — a deep groove in the stratum corneum — which extends from the undersurface of the callus. Beneath the cornoid plug the stratum granulosum layer is absent, whereas elsewhere it is well developed.
3. Moderate atrophy to complete absence of the stratum granulosum is one of the diagnostic histologic characteristics of this lesion. Also of paramount diagnostic significance is the hyperplasia and dilitation of the sweat gland units in the deeper portions of the dermis directly beneath the lesions.[132]

Differential Diagnosis

Differential diagnosis is not difficult either clinically or histologically. The tumor most similar is verruca plantaris, which bleeds after paring and is microscopically quite different from porokeratosis plantaris discreta.

Prognosis

Prognosis without treatment usually involves a prolonged, painful disability, although some podiatrists relate cases of spontaneous resolution. There are no reported cases of malignant transformation.

Treatment

Steinberg initially suggested that complete surgical extirpation was the best therapy for porokeratosis plantaris discreta. Most podiatrists advocate surgical correction of the bony part involved by any one of the multitude of procedures described in Volume II of this series. The surgical treatment of the IPK, with or without surgical removal of the tumor. Biomechanical evaluation has shown that rebalancing the weight bearing stresses of the foot can alleviate pain and often resolve the mass. Many podiatrists combine surgical and biomechanical correction for maximum insurance of resolution.

Dribbon, Baruch, and Weisfeld have described an intralesional injection of sclerosing solution: 1 ml. of 4% ethanol in 2% plain xylocaine, weekly for one to four weeks.[8,35,142] Favorable results are obtained by reduction of pain through the necrosis of sensory nerves in the area, and shrinkage of the hypertrophied gland by inflammation, necrosis, and fibrosis.

Note: The most outstanding feature about porokeratosis plantaris discreta is the paucity of literature regrading it. Certainly, more clinical and pathologic studies are needed before better preventive and corrective measures can be evaluated.

3. SEBACEOUS CYST (PILAR, WEN)

A cyst is a closed pouch or sac with a definite wall which contains fluid, semifluid, or solid material. There has been considerable debate in recent years among dermatopathologists as to whether a true *sebaceous* cyst even exists. Montgomery states that though the sebaceous cyst is clinically almost undistinguishable from the epidermal (inclusion) cyst, the sebaceous variety has a capsule of connective tissue, as opposed to epidermal tissue, and its cheesy, odoriferous contents are the break-down products of sebaceous sweat gland cells.[95] However, most authors seem to agree with Kligman that sebaceous cyst is a misnomer;[1,41,83,91,111] actually this tumor is a pilar cyst because its capsule is epidermal tissue and its contents are the products of incomplete keratinization of hair follicles.[78] It is often coextensive with the hair follicles.[23] Hence, the pilar cyst is just one variety of epidermal "keratinous" cyst. Pinkus, in 1969, states that sebaceous cysts are actually trichilemmal cysts.[105]

Pilar cysts comprise only one to fifteen percent of keratinous cysts,[41 91] over 90% of these pilar cysts occur on the scalp and about 9% occur on the back.[91] This particular cyst is very rare on the foot. Obviously, this cyst cannot develop on the palms and soles as there are no hair follicles (nor sebaceous glands) in these areas. All authors confirm this and a thorough review of the literature failed to yield a single reported case.

Allen states that the pilo-sebaceous cyst is most common on the face and back of adolescent patients with a background of acne vulgaris which is due to an increased activity of the sebaceous glands. Here again, differential diagnosis is difficult in that the most common sites for true epidermal cysts are the trunk and back. Pilar cysts often become inflammed and suppurative and approximately 1% to 4% appear to be pre-cancerous.[95]

4. EPIDERMAL INCLUSION CYST

Epidermal cysts are by far the most common of the "keratinous" cysts. They may arise primarily from rudimentary epithelial "rests"[95] or as a result of blocked hair follicles in which the epithelium of the epidermal lining undergoes an incomplete keratinization (rather than the hair itself contributing the keratinous material as in the pilar cyst).[91] Gross relates that these cysts are present in 1.2% of the population.[56]

Quite often epidermal cysts may be acquired by the "innoculation of a fragment of epidermis into the dermis following infection, an insect bite, a wound, a foreign body or other trauma,"[1] hence, the name "inclusion" cyst. Wein and Caro discussed traumatic epithelial cysts in 1934,[143] and Schultze described a hair as a foreign body in the sole of the foot in 1950.[117] Epidermal inclusion cysts of the foot are nearly always of the acquired type, frequently seen as a complication around the distal phalanx after nail surgery, and are not at all uncommon. Frequently, a history of having gone barefoot may be given as this significantly increases the incidence of trauma to the foot.

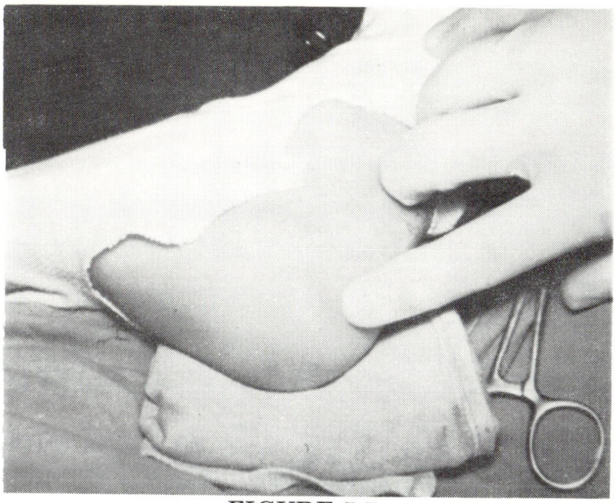

FIGURE 5-7

Epidermal Cyst: Epidermal cyst involving the posterior, plantar apex of the heel.

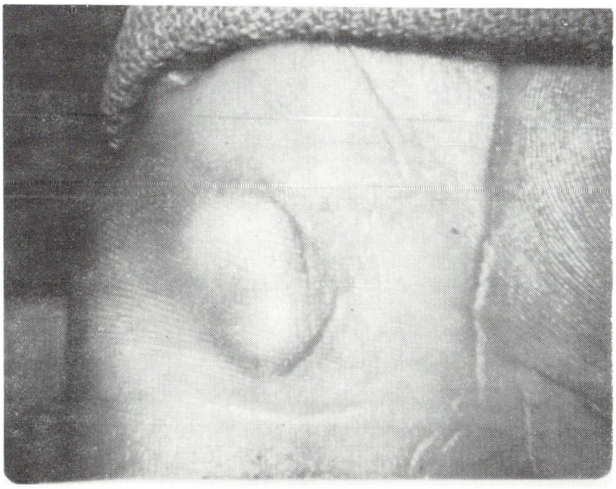

FIGURE 5-8

Epidermal Cyst: Epidermal cyst causing a large amount of soft tissue bulging on the plantar surface of the foot.

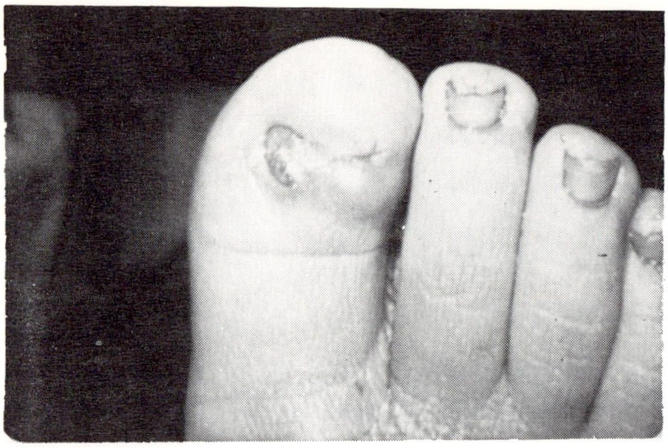

FIGURE 5-9

Epidermal Inclusion Cyst: Epidermal inclusion cyst of the nail bed, often a complication following nail surgery.

Clinical Considerations

Epidermal inclusion cysts of the foot are typically non-pigmented (usually whitish in color), semi-fluctuant tumors which may exist either superficially in the dermis or more deeply. They vary in shape and size from a few millimeters to several centimeters. They are generally asymptomatic unless there is an associated inflammatory reaction or the tumor is subject to pressure. These tumors occasionally grow rapidly and malignant progression has infrequently been reported.[95]

Review of the Literature

In 1957, Morrell reported a callus with an associated "pilonoidal" cyst of the sole secondary to the penetration of a dog hair.[96] In 1959, Silverman and Kove described an epidermal cyst at the site where the patient had stepped on a nail five years previous,[120] and Taub recorded an inclusion cyst of the heel with a foreign body reaction.[133] Maclin reported an epidermal inclusion cyst secondary to a wood splinter in 1965,[26] and Campbell described a large inclusion cyst which he excised from between the second and third metatarsals.[21] In 1971 Berlin reported three cases of epidermal inclusion cysts of the foot, none of which related a definite history of trauma, despite the presence of foreign body reaction histologically; however, trauma was believed to be the precipitating cause.[11] Recently, Dix reported an inclusion cyst following osteotripsy.[34] Greer reported a case involving the plantar surface and states they are rare.[50] We believe it is just the contrary and they are not reported because of insignificant findings.

Histopathology

The cyst usually exists in the dermis. It is lined with keratinizing epidermis which casts off horny cells that do not have typically rigid cell membranes; these fragile cells liberate incompletely keratinized, horny contents into the cystic space.[78]

In the acquired type there is often an accompanying foreign body reaction, consisting of a lymphocytic and giant cell infiltration, and there may be scar tissue present. If the cyst exists in a weight bearing area, overlying hyperkeratotic tissue may be seen.

Differential Diagnosis

Differential diagnosis may be made clinically, but must be confirmed histopathologically. It includes: ganglionic cyst, fibroma, lipoma, dermatofibroma, verrucae plantaris, porokeratosis plantaris discreta, eccrine poroma, nevus fibroma, plantar fibromatosis.

Treatment

Needle aspiration of an epidermal cyst may yield a whitish, semi-fluid to cheesy material which is the broken down keratin contained in the cyst. Complications from this technique can develop into ulceration as has been experienced by the authors. This rarely affects a cure because the epidermal capsule of the tumor proliferated this material as before.

Excision en toto is nearly always curative provided that the entire capsule and the foreign body, if present, are excised.

Complications

Recurrence occurs frequently because any fragment of the epidermal capsule or keratinous contents of the cyst which may remain after excision can initiate the reformation of the entire cyst.

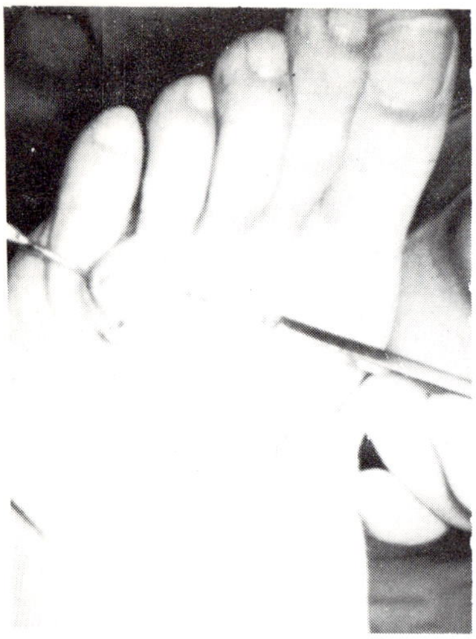

FIGURE 5-14

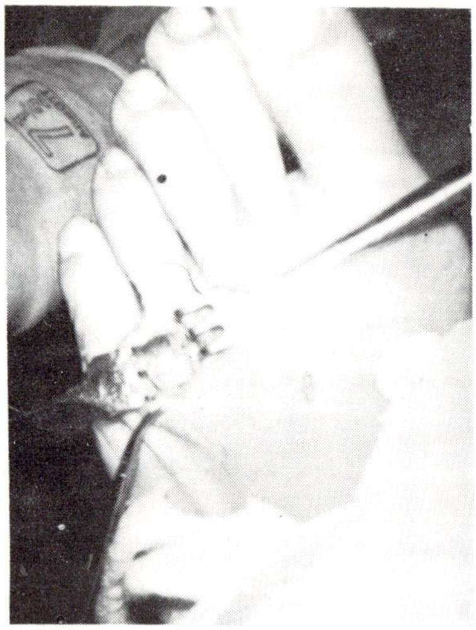

FIGURE 5-15

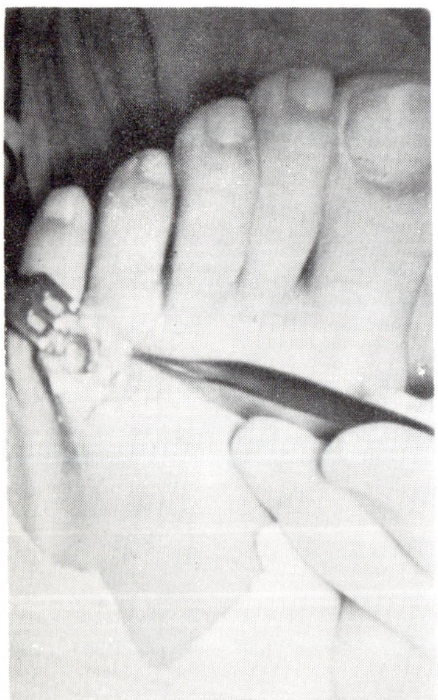

FIGURE 5-16

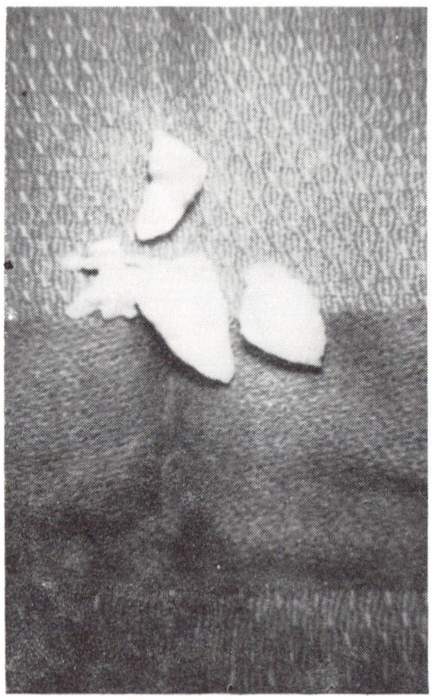

FIGURE 5-17

Epidermal Inclusion Cyst: A large epidermal inclusion cyst containing specific cystic sections. Previous symptoms revealed a painful plantar callous. The skin lesion disappeared after surgery.

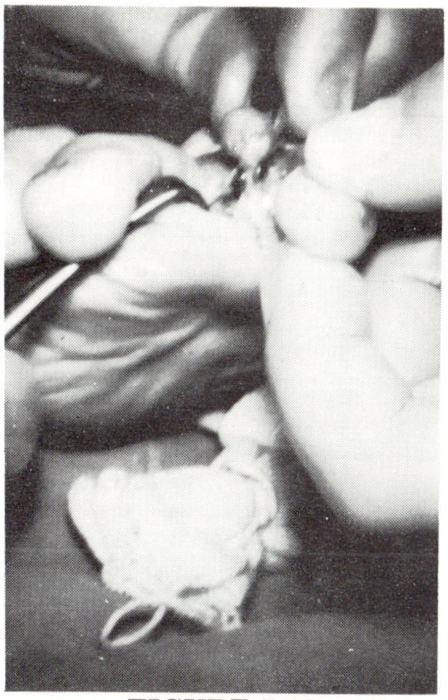

FIGURE 5-10

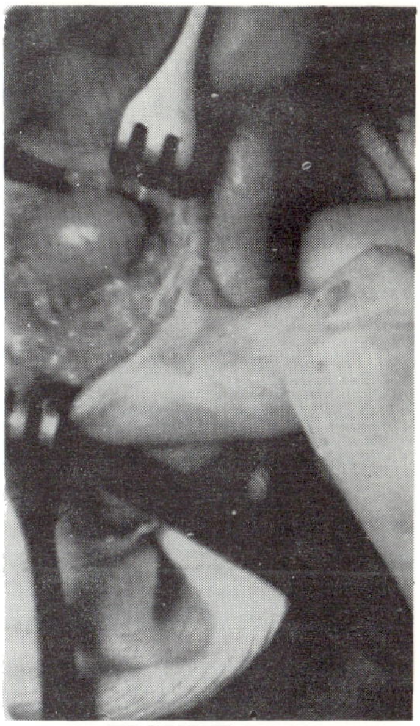

FIGURE 5-11

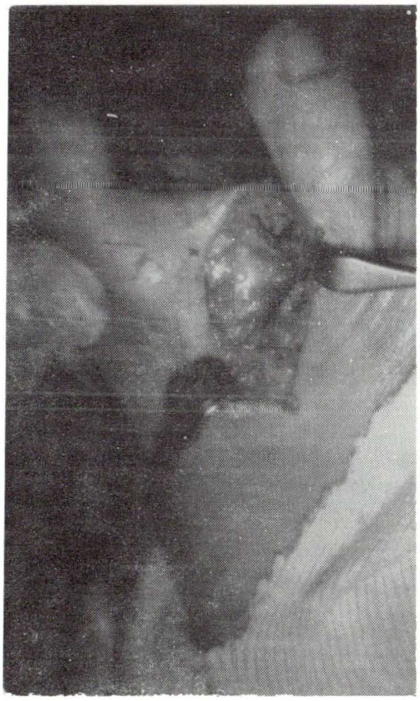

FIGURE 5-12

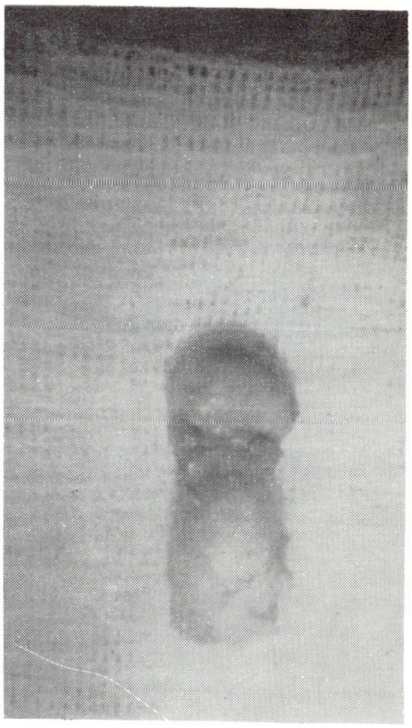

FIGURE 5-13

Epidermal Inclusion Cyst: A large intermetatarsal epidermal inclusion cyst undergoing surgical excision, cystic portions have completely solidified, previous history showed a giant cell tumor had been removed seven years previous to this surgery.

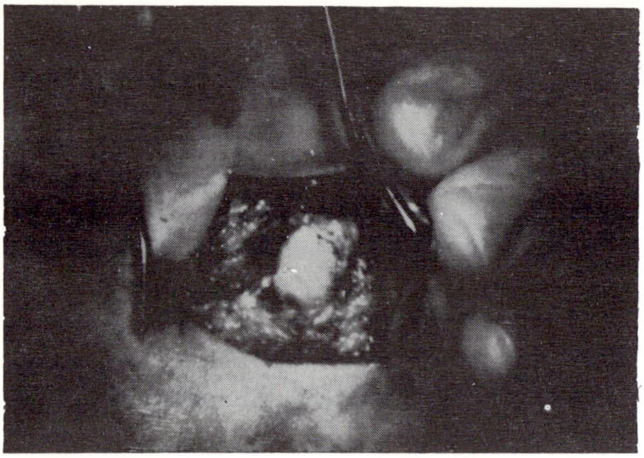

FIGURE 5-18

Epidermal Inclusion Cyst: Surgical exposure revealing large cyst under the first metatarsal head. These lesions can occur anywhere on the foot.

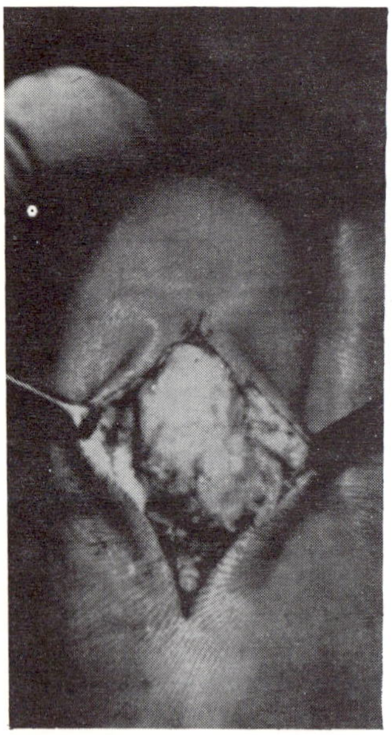

FIGURE 5-19

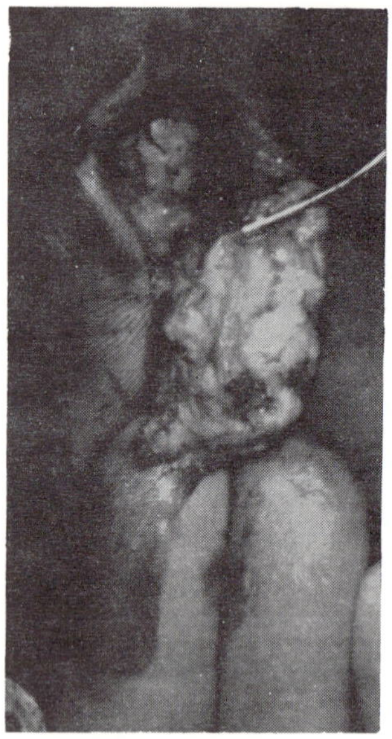

FIGURE 5-20

Epidermal Inclusion Cyst: A large an irregular lesion undergoing surgical excision on the hallux toe.

Fibrous Tumors

1. FIBROMA (INOMA)

A fibroma is a benign neoplasm derived from fibrous connective tissue and is more commonly seen in association with other tissue structures. It is rarely seen in a pure state involving the foot except in the regions of the pedal skin.

Clinical Picture

Fibroma may take place at any age and appear in any site with a tendency to occur in the connective tissue sheaths of nerves, sheaths of muscle fascia, periosteum of bones and dermal connective tissue. Fibromas are usually small, ranging in size from 1-4 cm, encapsulated and appearing as spherical to ovoid nodules. They are usually of a firm consistency varying from a soft rubbery pliable mass (fibroma molle) to a very hard nodule (fibroma durum). Grossly, the capsule is usually apparent.

Histopathology

Microscopically, it may give an appearance of a firm white glistening surface usually absent from necrosis and hemorrhage. There is evidence of spindle shaped fibrocytes and fibroblasts which have elongated nuclei. There are finely divided chromatin and long tapering cytoplasmic processes on either end. The cells are either in random alignment or in a large wavy ribbon of parallel bundles of cells. Metatasis is rare and anaplasia is absent. Between the fibroblasts are varying amounts of collagen which gives the tumor its firm consistency.

Prognosis

Usually there is no problem with this tumor except for occasional pain due to the pressure on nerves and rarely, if ever, are malignant changes seen.

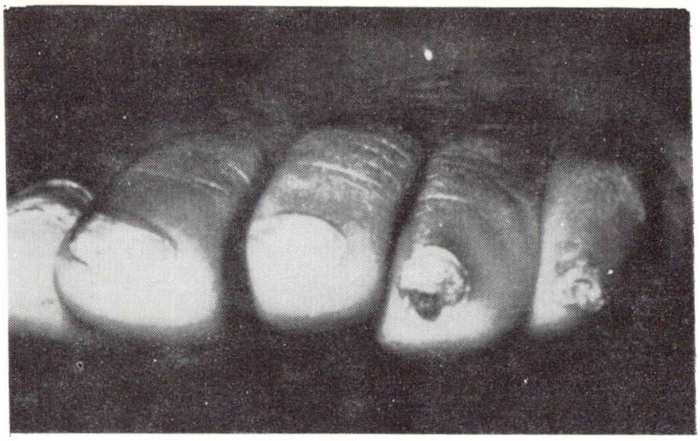

FIGURE 5-21

Subungual Fibroma: These lesions are often asymptomatic and often bleed in trimming ones toe nails.

Treatment

Simple excision is the treatment of choice. Electrocautery and curettement may be utilized in treating small lesions. Larger lesions involving the pedal skin may need skin grafting.

2. PERIUNGUAL FIBROMA

Periungual fibroma is a fibroma which involves the nail fold.

Etiology

No definite etiologic factor has been established. These tumors are associated findings in tuberous sclerosis, von Recklinghausen's disease and traumatic factors. The authors have even seen these lesions occuring as a result of trauma from nail surgery.

Review of the Literature

The medical literature is not overflowing with cases of periungual fibromas of the feet. Some authors in fact, when reporting periungual fibromas do not differentiate between lesions of the fingers or toes, but simply report the incidence as to sex, age, etc. Periungual fibromas were first described by Kothe in 1903.[80] Serger and Wendleberger, in 1920, described tuberous sclerosis

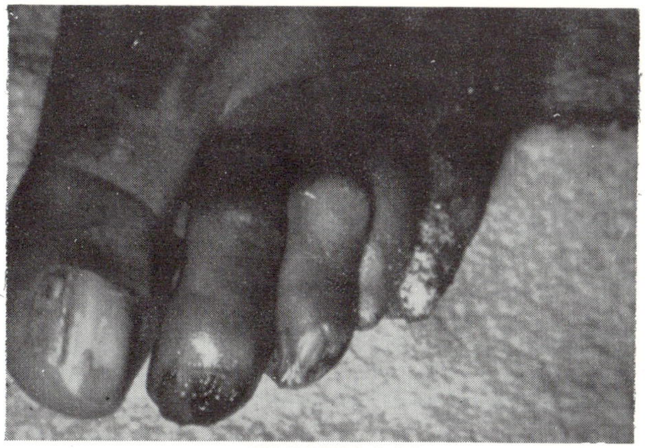

FIGURE 5-22

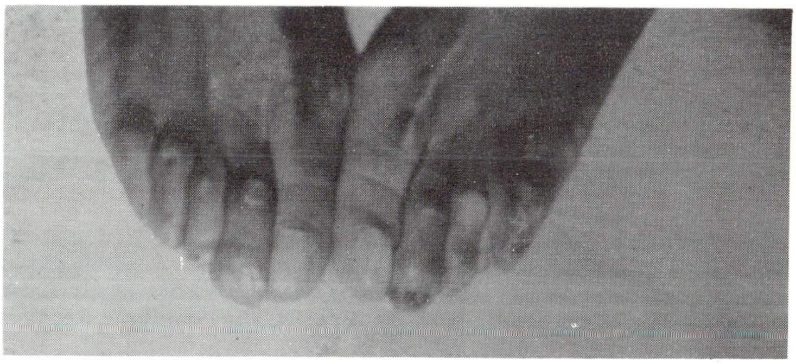

FIGURE 5-23

Periungual Fibroma: The above photos reveal periungual fibromas involving all nail bed areas. As many as six lesions were noted on a single side of one nail.

with fibromatous tumors in a thirty-one year old male. In 1931, J. Busch reported finding more lesions on the toenails than on the digits of the hand.[20] He suggested that pressure from shoes might have been a stimulus for the formation of these fibromas. King-Smith, in 1932, described adenoma sebaceum with nevoid growths about the toenail and thought them to be congenital. Montfer, in 1933, described papillomas of the nail bed in a twenty-seven year old patient with a possible combination of tuberous sclerosis and neurofibromatosis. Kurtz, in 1934, described a case of tuberous sclerosis with fibromatosis changes of the nail bed. Oulmann, in 1935, described fibrous warts on all the toenails of a twenty-two year old male with adenoma sebaceum. Stout in 1954 suggested that a differential diagnosis must be made from the ungual fibromas of tuberous sclerosis which are multiple and tend to recur, from that of juvenile fibromatosis.[26] He proposed that this brought up the question of whether patients with acquired digital fibrokeratoma have abortive tuberous sclerosis.

Histopathology

According to Mihregan, who described recurring digital fibrous tumors of childhood, these growths are ". . . .covered by a layer of slightly acanthotic epidermis. The tumor replaced the corium from immediately below the basal layer of the epidermis and extended into the subcutaneous fat tissue. The growth consisted of a proliferation of spindle-shaped fibroblast collagen bundles, and small capillary blood vessels. The fibroblasts had elongated or stellate nuclei and ill-defined cytoplasm and were surrounded by intersecting bundles of collagen. Occasionally, small pieces of elastic fibers were present in different areas. . .

The most interesting and characteristic histopathologic feature of this tumor was the presence within the cytoplasm of some fibroblasts of small, round or ovoid bodies ranging from three microns to ten microns in diameter. . ."[92]

Clinical Picture

Feinstein described these periungual fibromas as being "the most consistent finding associated with tuberous sclerosis on the foot. . . These occur after puberty, and are firm, smooth, flesh-colored tumors protruding from under the nail folds."[39] They are all small in size and to those unfamiliar with the lesions, they may appear to be periungual verruca. Periungual fibroma associated with tuberous sclerosis are referred to as Kernan's tumors. However, these lesions may present themselves with no underlying systemic relationship.

Treatment

Although these lesions may bother some patients because of their cosmetic appearance, they are not, by themsleves, symptomatic, and therefore, no treatment is necessary. Excision of

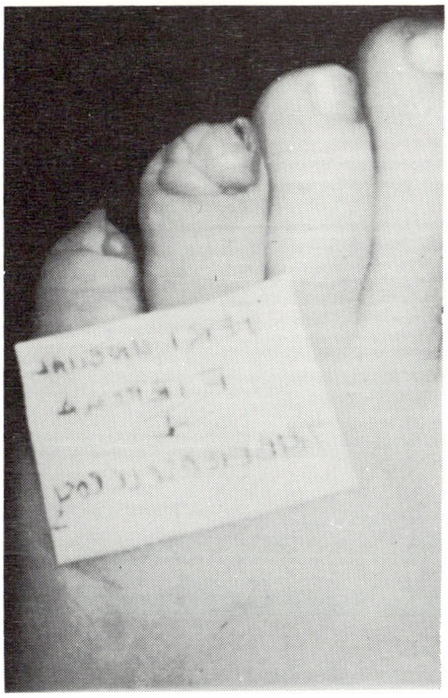

FIGURE 5-24

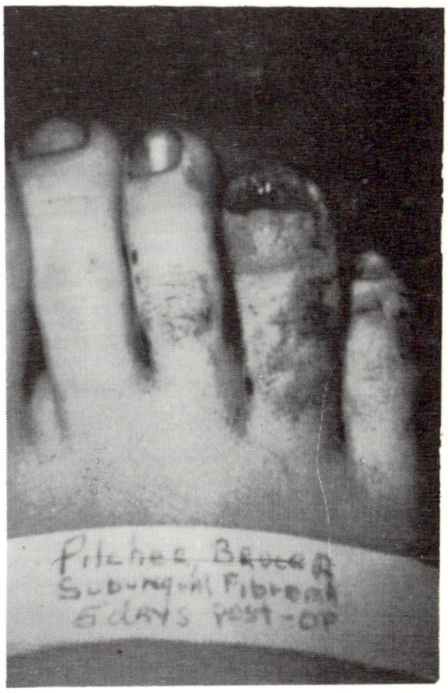

FIGURE 5-25

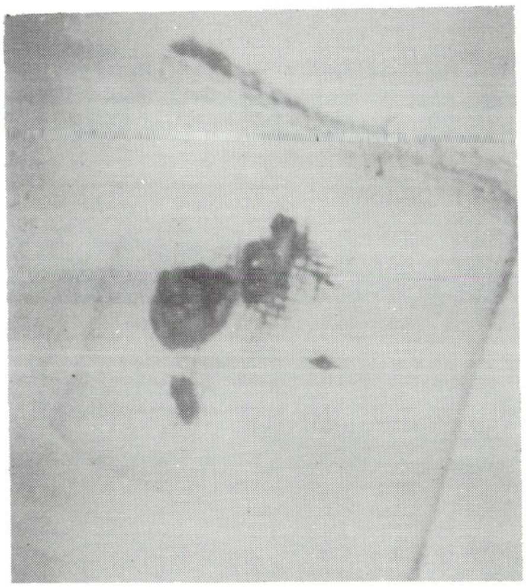

FIGURE 5-26

Periungual Fibroma: Periungual fibromas are very frequently associated with tuberoslerosis and Von Recklinghausen's disease. Radical nail bed excision and matrixsectomy are necessary for surgical cure.

these lesions should be performed if symptomatic or for histological diagnosis. Since these lesions have a high recurrence rate, radical excision of the tumor and surrounding nail bed and matrix should be performed.

3. RECURRENT DIGITAL FIBROMA OF CHILDHOOD

Recurrent digital fibroma is a benign tumor found in childhood. Its location is limited to the fingers and toes and it is present at birth or develops usually before the age of five. In 1965, Reye discovered the presence of intracytoplasmotic inclusion-like bodies which are highly specific in distinguishing this lesion from other fibromatous tumors in childhood. It was Reye who initiated the name "recurring digital fibrous tumors of childhood." Previously it was known as dermatofibroma, neurofibroma, sarcoma, dermal fibromatosis, infantile digital fibromatosis or infantile dermal fibromatosis. Initially, Jensen suggested the cause to be viral and was later supported by Reye with his demonstration of cellular inclusion bodies. It wasn't until 1971, however, when Battefora and Hines confirmed the viral origin of the condition with their electron microscopic studies. They found amorphous and fibrillary inclusions with an appearance similar to that of viroplasm of fibroblasts infected with Shope fibroma virus.

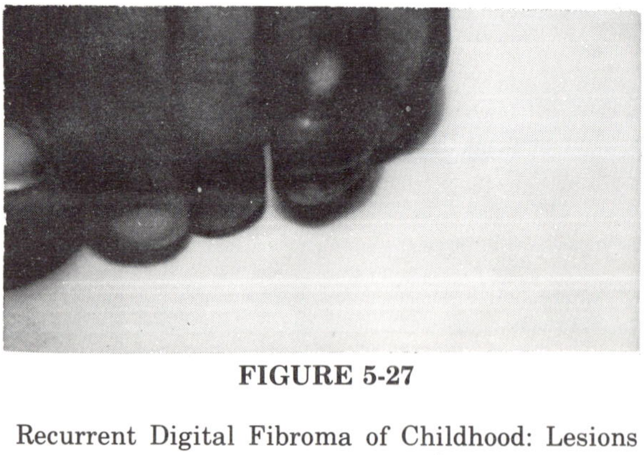

FIGURE 5-27

Recurrent Digital Fibroma of Childhood: Lesions often asymptomatic, surgical excision often require skin grafting. (Courtesy of Adolph Galinsky, D.P.M., Chicago, Illinois.)

One reason for its infrequent occurrence in the literature is that it is often misdiagnosed. The hemotoxylin and eosin stains often do not demonstrate the inclusion cytoplasmic bodies. Another factor is that this tumor may be misdiagnosed as a fibrosarcoma because of its frequent recurrence. The high incidence of recurrence is believed to be due to its irregular borders or to the appearance of small segments distant to the main growth. The growth rate is normally slow.

Treatment

Best results are obtained by taking the widest possible excision without damaging the function of the digit. Sometimes excision with the employment of a skin graft has been used. Amputation should be the ultimate last choice.

4. DERMATOFIBROMA (HISTIOCYTOMA, SCLEROSING HEMANGIOMA)

Today the terms histiocytoma and dermatofibroma are often used interchangeably. They are frequently seen on the dorsum and uncommon on the plantar surface of the foot. Other names given to describe this tumor are sclerosing hemangioma, cutaneous nodule, dermatofibroma lenticulare, fibroma simplex, xanthofibroma, or just fibroma.[28 41] The term dermatofibroma was first used in 1930 by Schreus in describing a tumor, while the name histiocytoma cutis was introduced by Senear and Caro.[28 98] At one time the tumors were thought to be separate entities which some authorities still believe, but the general opinion today is to group the types under one heading.[28,98,108]

Histiocytoma cutis is the common term used to indicate certain benign dermal fibrous tumors composed of blood vessels, fibrous tissue, histiocytes and inflammatory cells of different sizes. Niemi states that both are composed of fibroblasts and collagen fibers, but, in addition a histiocytoma may contain histiocytes with a foamy cytoplasm and it may be possibly pigmented and have the capability to phagocytose. The fibroblast of the dermatofibroma contained a cell with an oval, often short and thick nucleus. In differentiating the fibroblast, the histiocytoma con-

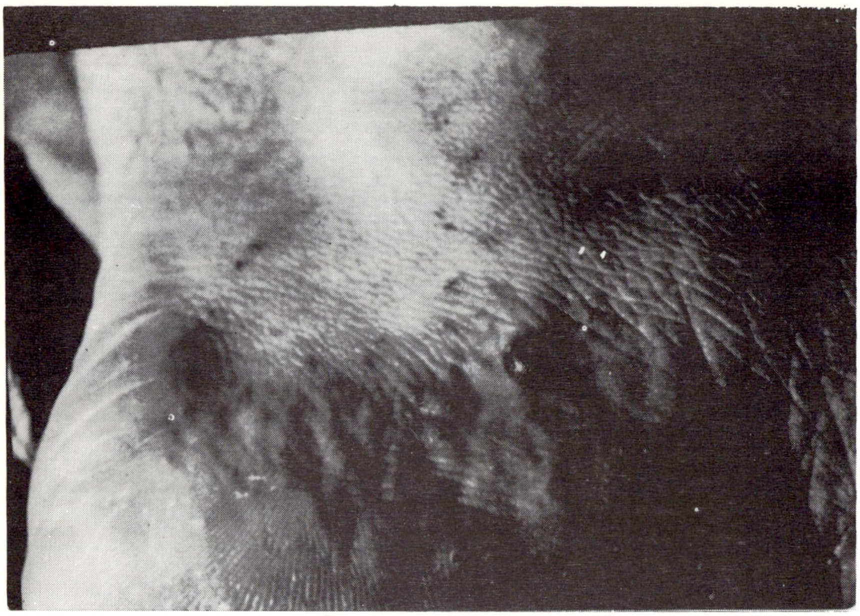

FIGURE 5-28

Histiocytoma: Dark, firm lesion often asymptomatic, medial border of the foot. (Courtesy of J. V. Ganley, D.P.M., Norristown, Pa.)

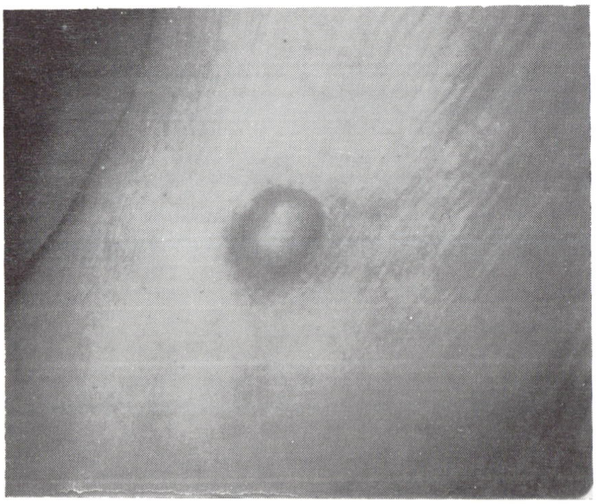

FIGURE 5-29

Dermatofibroma: Large dermatofibroma in region of foot and ankle.

tained intracytoplasmic bodies which were in the form of foam or pigments. Hyperkeratosis and epidermal acanthosis was common in both, but the dermatofibroma demonstrated an increase in the pigmentation of the basal cells of the epidermis. Clinically Niemi stated that dermatofibroma was more prevalent all over the body, being more frequent on the upper limbs, while the histiocytoma appeared more frequently on the lower limb.

Clinical Appearance

It is a firm tumor of various connective tissue elements which probably develop as a result of some type of inflammatory process. A number of authorities believe that the tumors arise from a vascular origin which transform from a highly vascularized lesion to a solid cellular tumor.[54 73 109] The theory adhered to states that there is a succession of phases which tends to obliterate a capillary angioma. Repeated hemorrhage from the malformed vessels is said to be the initiating factor which causes a proliferative cellular response of endothelial cells and connective tissue stroma resulting in a pigmented cytoscleral reaction. The reason for the controversy in nomenclature is that histiologically there are three basic patterns. One is that of numerous fibrous tissue, giving rise to the name dermatofibroma. Another is described as a vascular tumor with variable degrees of reactive fibrous obliteration of the vessels and named sclerosing hemangioma. Finally it is called a histiocytoma because of the many active histiocytes.[123]

They usually appear as hard single nodules, but may be multiple. They vary in color depending on their vascularity, lipid and hemosiderin content from a red-blue to yellow and then to brown or black. They are frequently of long duration and grow slowly. The tumors are well defined, not encapsulated, and vary in size. Most are painless, although some may cause pain due to ulceration and bleeding, or may become infected. The histiocytoma cutis must be differentiated from a malignant melanoma, synovial cyst, inclusion cyst, foreign body granuloma, granuloma pyogenicum, and fibrosarcoma. In the subungual area other differential diagnosis includes the fibromas seen in epiloia and even keratoacanthoma.

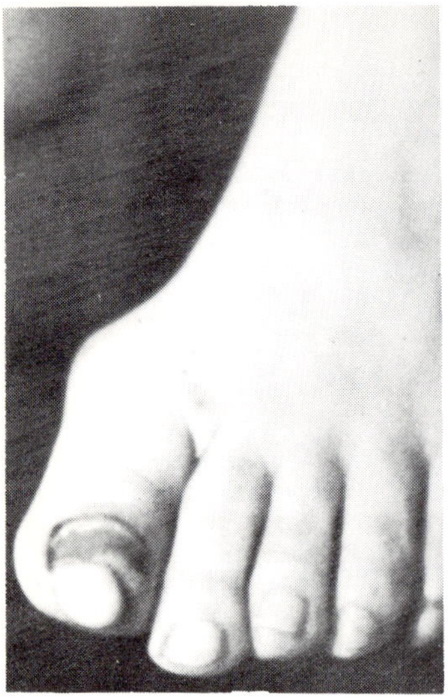

FIGURE 5-30

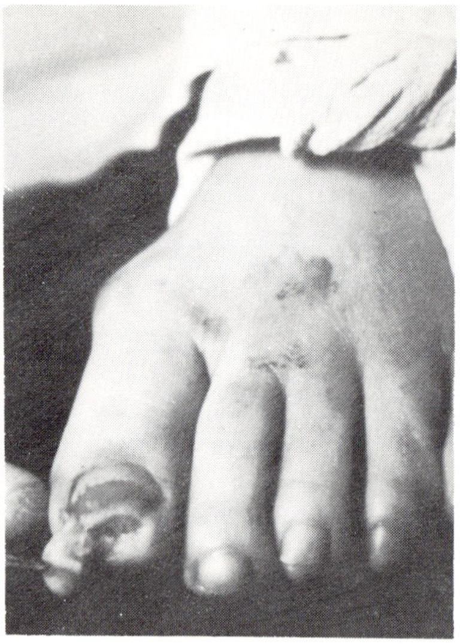

FIGURE 5-31

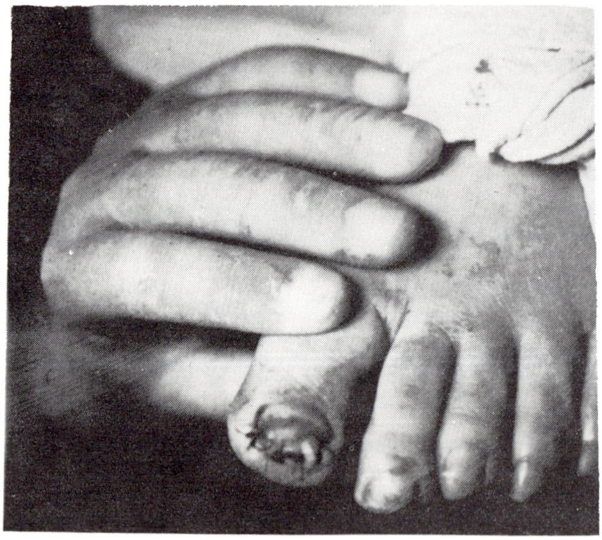

FIGURE 5-32

Dermatofibroma: Surgical excision of a lesion at the distal aspect of the toe. Any lesion involving nail bed area. Removal of the nail is necessary prior to excision.

Onset

The tumors are more prevalent in early adulthood and rare in childhood. One case was reported in a baby 10 days after delivery, in which the lesion presented itself as a swelling on the second toe of the left foot.[123]

Histology

The majority of the tumors occur within the dermal and subcutaneous tissues. Sometimes they may become elevated or even pedunculated. On section they appear as solid, poorly limited areas, no true encapsulation exists and pseudopod-like extensions may project into adjacent tissue spaces. They vary in color from black to purple, red or yellow depending on the vascularity, lipid and hemosiderin content. The lesion is usually not larger than 2-3 cm in diameter. Usually there are tightly whorled and interlocking bundles of spindle cells. Within the whorls there appear vascular channels which are almost completely obliterated. The bundles and whorls are arranged in a stellate, radiating or in any other small complex design. The cells appear uniform in size and shape. In some areas the tumors may be collagenous, in others it may exhibit old hemmorhage and hemosiderin pigmentation while in still others large foreign body type giant cells may be present. Often, foam cells and Touton giant cells are scattered in clusters or small islands within a histiocytoma. When foam cells form large groups, the lesion acquires a xanthomatous appearance. On occasion it may resemble dermatofibrosarcoma protuberans, but the cells do not metastasize and mitotic activity is minimal or absent.

Treatment

Treatment usually consists of complete excision of the lesion.

5. KELOIDS AND HYPERTROPHIC SCARS

The term keloid is derived from the Greek word "cheloids", meaning crab's claw. A keloid was first described and named by Alibert in 1806, in which he termed it "les cancroides".[26,79,128,146] In 1817 he changed the name to cheloides, because of the resemblance to shell fish, with its process like projections implanted in

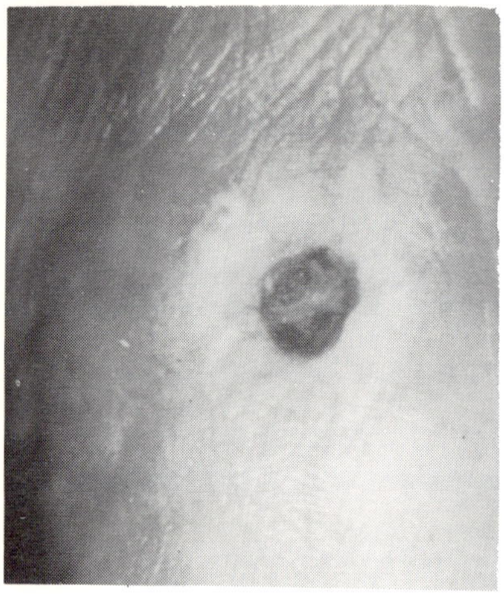

FIGURE 5-33

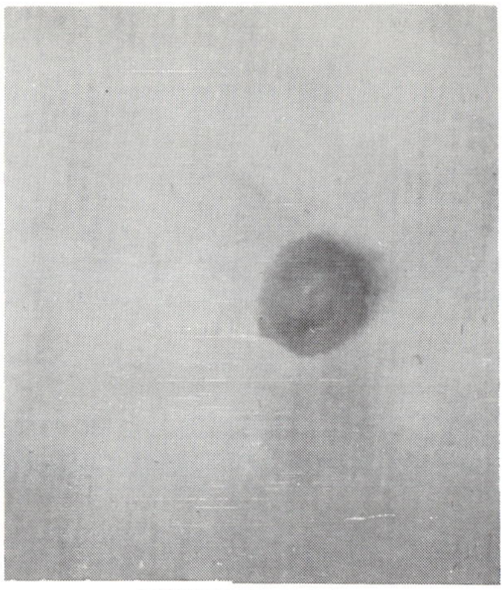

FIGURE 5-34

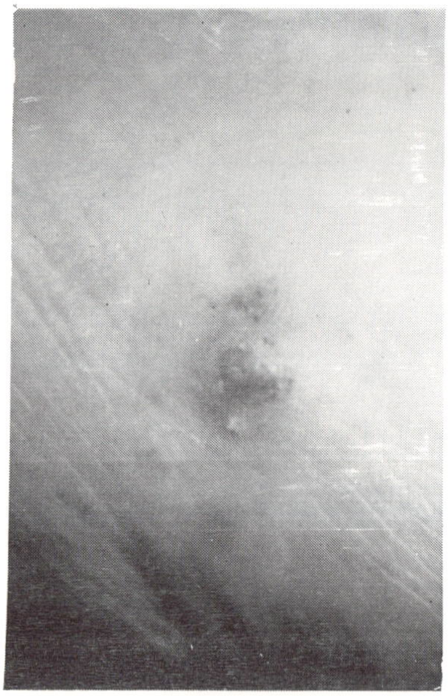

FIGURE 5-35

Dermatofibroma: Dermatofibroma involving plantar surfaces of the foot are uncommon. Blunt disection and electrocautery have been employed with this lesion.

the skin. In 1854, the term keloid, which meant a mark or blemish, was introduced by Addison, although he was describing scleroderma.[79] Addison classified two types, one being the spontaneous or true, and the other being cicatrical. Having classified two types, a controversy was started in the years to come to differentiate a keloid from a hypertrophic scar.

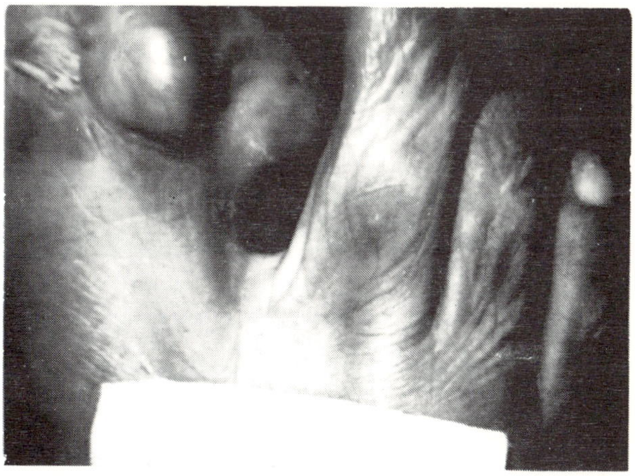

FIGURE 5 36

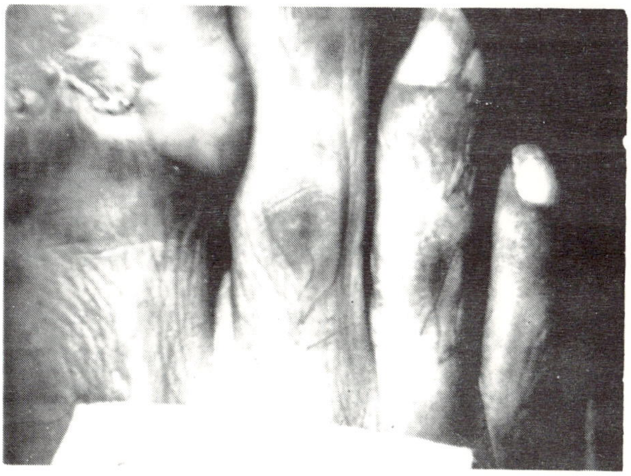

FIGURE 5-37

Keloid: Large bulbous keloid resulting from prior nail surgery.

Etiology

There has been no precise definition or etiology for the formation of either keloids or hypertrophic scars, but rather a number of theories. For our purposes, a keloid is described as a scar extending beyond the original wound and a hypertrophic scar being one which remains within the boundaries of the original wound; both are elevated above the skin. Most authorities agree that local trauma to the dermis is the precipitating factor causing the scar formation.[61 79, 127 134]

There are other possible causes which tend to form excessive scars. A foreign body reaction, due to inclusion of tissue or outside material which stimulated fibrous tissue proliferation.[128 136] The amount of scar formation in a wound varies according to whether the wound heals by first or second intention.[84, 128] Hematoma formation, infection, devitalized tissues, dressing methods and wound closure all contribute to the amount of scar formed. Wounds which heal with too much tension, or the placing of sutures too tightly, may influence scar formation. Of course sur-

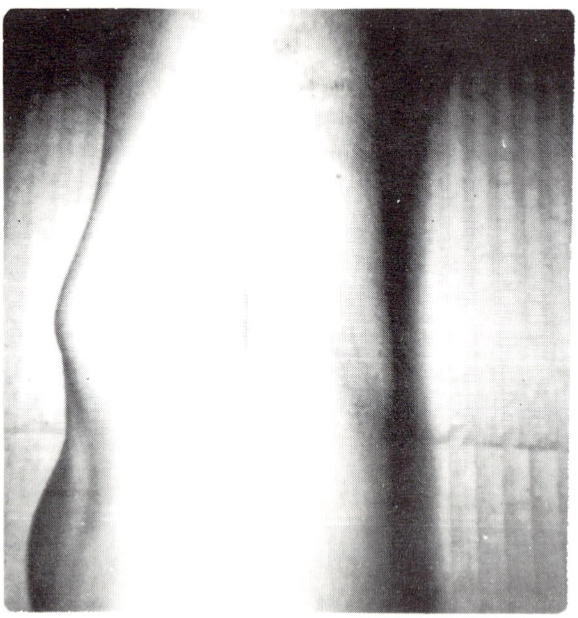

FIGURE 5-38

Hypertrophic Scar: Hypertrophic scar extensor surface of foot and ankle.

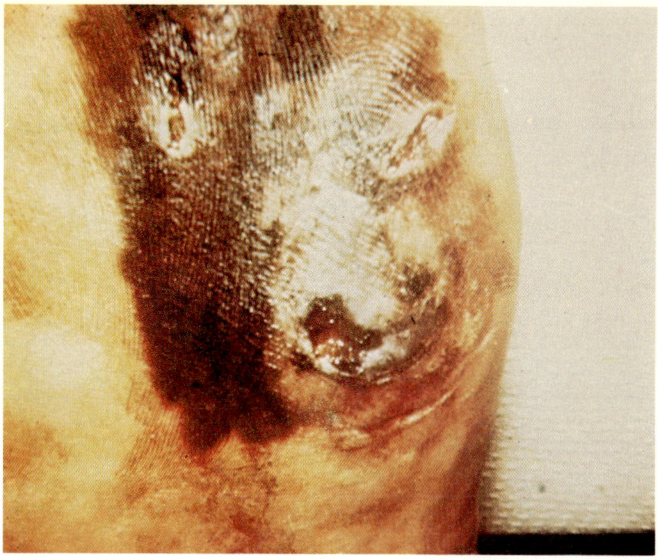

Malignant Melanoma — A large ulcerative melanoma of the sole.

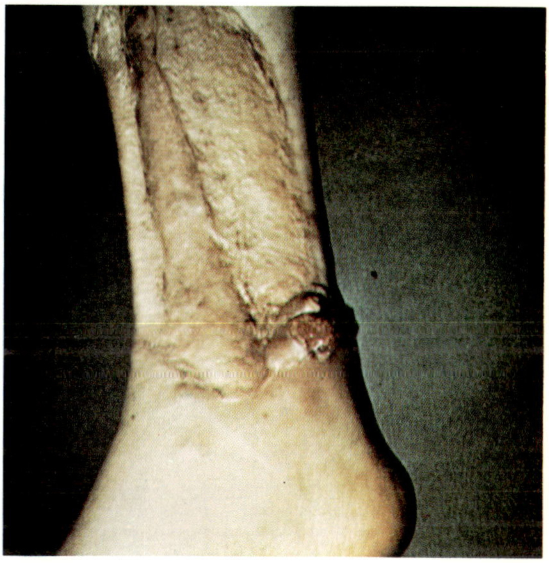

Melanoma—Recurrent melanoma in graft site. (Courtesy of Ronald Goldner, M.D. Baltimore, Maryland.)

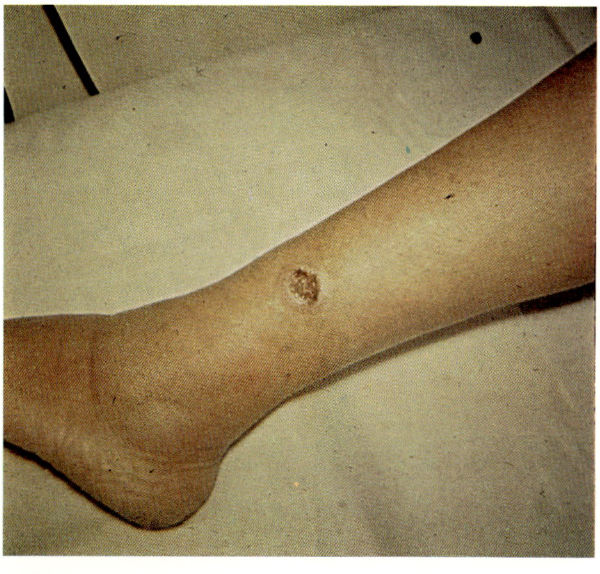

Basal Cell Carcinoma — (Lower Leg) Probably the least common of the skin malignancies seen on the foot. (Courtesy of Isidore Zeligman, M.D., Baltimore, Maryland.)

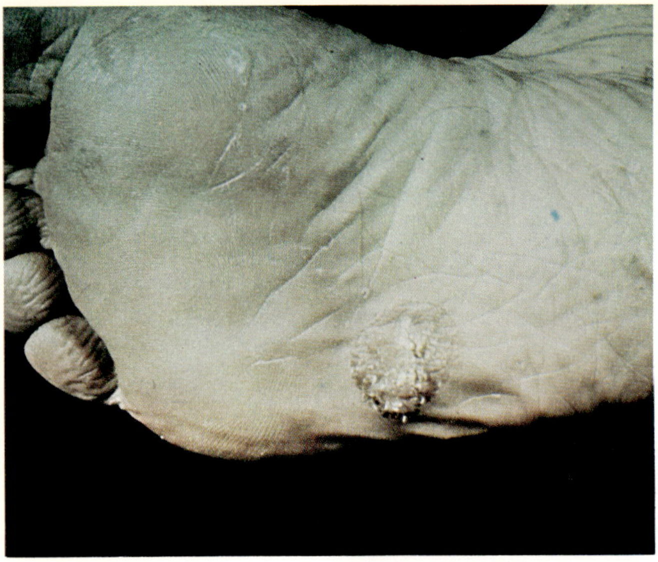

Bowens' Disease — Reveals dull red patch with sharp but irregular outline and moderate hyperkeratosis due to plantar weight bearing pressures. (Courtesy of Ronald Goldner, M.D., Baltimore, Maryland.)

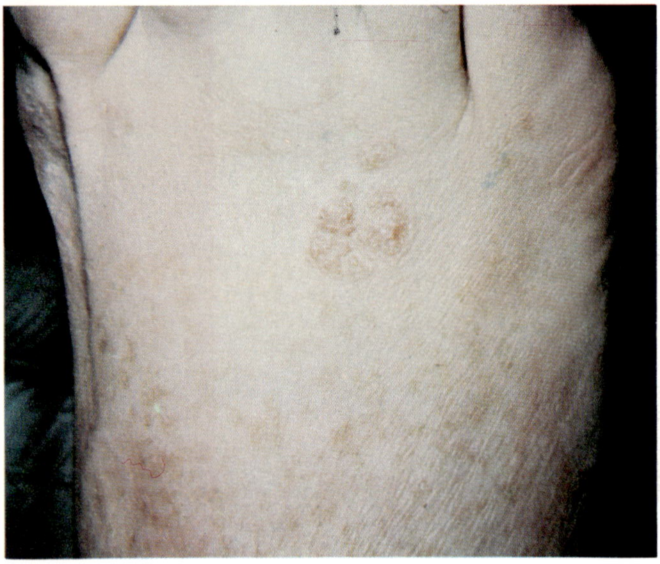

Bowens' Disease — Superficial crusting has been removed from the lesions. Hyperkeratosis may occur on dorsal surfaces of the foot usually initiated from shoe pressure.

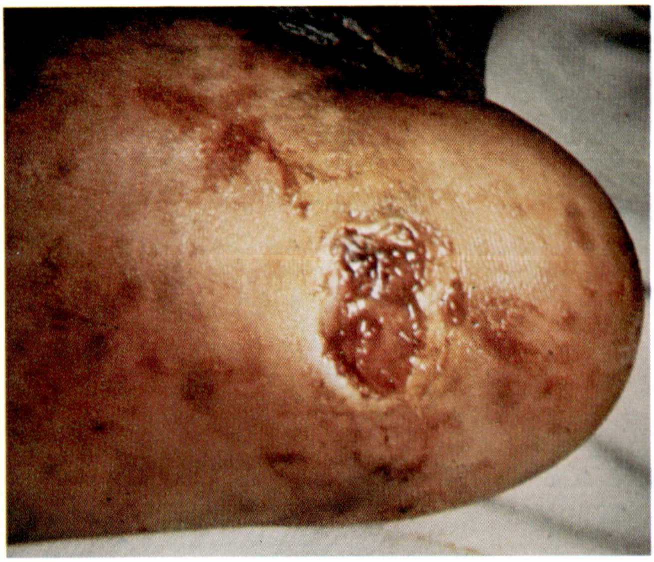

Squamous Cell Carcinoma — On the heel, malignant lesions may develop at the site of prior x-irradiation, or from pre-existing arsenical keratosis. (Courtesy of William V. R. Shellow, M.D., Los Angeles, California.)

gical technique is very important; injury through mishandling of the tissue, or improper placement of incisions in relation to the skin lines of tension such as cutting across flexion creases. Incisions that cross joints tend to spread and the muscle pull on the wound will continually stimulate fibroblastic activity. Scar formation varies in different parts of the body with the lower extremity being more prone to suture marks; however the feet show little likelihood for keloid formation. The most common areas for keloid formation are the face, neck, ears, presternum, and deltoid region. There is definitely more of an incidence of keloids in dark-skinned individuals. It is believed that melanin may play a part by being more reactive to melanin stimulating hormone, but this has not been proven. Scars seem to appear where the melanin is more concentrated, such as in the face and neck, and not the palms and soles. Hormone activity also seems to be involved with scar formation, occurring with a hyperactive pituitary, being more common in puberty, pregnancy, and acromegaly. It is also a feature of Addison's Disease and hyperthyroidism.[79, 127] Keloids seem to be more prevalent in younger ages, and there seems to be an hereditary factor involved, although no good study has been done to prove this. Scar formation varies with age in the same individual. Therefore, one can conclude that there is no one cause, not every dark-skinned individual develops a keloid, and it may be a conglomerate of many factors. Peacock has theorized that the excessive scar formation is due to collagen metabolism.[101] He believes that at seven weeks of scar maturation, there should be an equilibrium of collagen synthesis and collagenolytic activity. If the collagenolytic activity is faulty, the scar formation will persist for a number of years and become excessive.

Most authorities are not in accord in listing certain characteristics to differentiate keloids from hypertrophic scars.[13,27,30,48,61,127,128,144] It is generally agreed that keloids seem to send pseudopod-like extensions into the adjacent healthy tissue extending beyond the boundries of the wound area. A hypertrophic scar remains within the wound area. Keloids seem to be more common in Negroes and dark-skinned people while hypertrophic scars seem to occur equally in both blacks and whites. A keloid is usually larger and firmer than a hypertrophic scar or false keloid. Keloids tend to grow gradually and don't regress spontaneously. They often have a tendency to recur following excision. Initially, both types of scars may produce itching or paresthesia and are easily traumatized, causing pain and burning sensation. In their immature state they are vascularized and red in color, gradually changing to a brownish leathery appearance before assuming its poorly vascularized to avascular firm white appearance which may be asymptomatic. Peacock differentiates the two by observing the amount of scar formation.[101] He believes the larger formation is a keloid and the lesser amount a hypertrophic scar. He feels that all clinical findings are arbitrary with the biological difference being one of quantity. Both scars are delayed in appearing, usually after normal healing has occurred at four to five weeks. Peacock uses the term 'overflow' to differentiate hypertrophic scar from keloid. 'Overflow' means that newly synthesized collagen has developed so quickly that the scar becomes pedunculated, inferring that in some scars, the mass of scar tissue is many times the size of what should appear as a normal scar.

Histology

There are many authoritative people who state unequivocably that there is a definite difference, histologically, between hypertrophic scars and keloids.[15,48,128,134] There are just as many authorities who take the opposite opinion that there is no difference.[26,36,63,87,101] The keloids and hypertrophic scars may be defined as benign cutaneous soft tissue tumors which are comprised of thick hyalinized collagen bundles, containing fibroblasts and blood vessels which are located in the subpapillary layer of the dermis. As stated before, hypertrophic scars remain confined to the area of the skin incision or injury, while the keloid tends to invade the surrounding tissues. Also, hypertrophic scars continue to grow for several weeks or months, then become inactive and tend to regress. Keloids continue to grow into bizarre forms which do not regress. Keloids and hypertrophic scars are classified under the heading of fibroma. Under the microscope it is difficult to distinguish the three; collagen is the constituent used often, but not always, to differentiate.[61,128] Collagen is the most important factor in scar formation. The kind and amount of collagen formed will determine the kind and amount of scar produced. In a keloid, the collagen fibers are arranged in nodular masses which extend and grow irregularly into the surrounding dermis and subcutaneous tissue where they blend into the surrounding normal collagen. A hypertrophic scar somewhat resembles a keloid in which the collagen fibers blend with the surrounding normal collagen fibers at the periphery, but the fibers also grow more uniformly and tend to lie parallel to the lines of force across the scar. In a fibroma, the collagen fibers are normal, containing a capsule preventing the blending of the collagen fibers with the surrounding tissues.

There are four stages which occur in the healing process. The first is the traumatic inflammatory stage which consists of local inflammation with capillary dilation and edema. The edges of the wound are kept close to each other by a fibrin clot which forms during the first three days after the injury. The destructive phase is next which occurs from the fourth to the sixth day consisting of the necrotic tissue being broken down and removed by invading leukocytes and macrophages. The proliferative phase follows in which new capillaries form which is believed to be stimulated by a chemotrophic effect causing substances to be liberated in the wound. As the capillaries begin to grow into the wound, the fibroblasts grow along the capillaries in a perivascular pattern. Collagen is formed and over a period of time the cell to collagen fiber ratio decreases while the tensile strength of the wound begins to increase. Finally, in the maturation phase, fibroplasia reaches its peak at about 14-21 days and wound shrinkage and maturation of the connective tissue in the wound begins. There is a decrease in the number of blood vessels and number of fibroblastic cells. Full maturity of the wound and, in particular, the collagen component of scar tissues, takes many months. The scar thickens and shows disarrangement of the collagen bundles.

The early stages of keloid and hypertrophic scar formation have been reported as being identical to normal healing.[15,27,144] In the latter stages, the reactive connective tissue elements either regress forming a normal scar, continue to proliferate, but along normal lines forming a hypertrophic scar, or undergo abnormal proliferation, forming a keloid. It has been shown that human scar tissue contains active collagen many months after healing appears clinically complete. The collagen synthesis and breakdown remains active for a long period of time in wound healing. The breakdown is usually achieved at about six weeks. In keloids, the cycle formation is similar to normal healing, but may be lengthened to months or years.

If one were to look under a microscope at a mature keloid and some hypertrophic scars, he would describe it as containing thick homogenous eosinophilic bands of collagen, intermingled with thin collagenous fibers and large active fibroblasts. The lesion occupies the dermis with the sweat glands, sebaceous glands, hair follicles, and arrectore pilorum being atrophic, destroyed or displaced by the scar. Elastic fibers are diminished or absent.

In the past, keloids were classified as pre-malignant, but they should not be. Only two cases were ever reported as malignant and one was in 1888.[64]

For those who believe that there is a difference between hypertrophic scars and keloids histologically, below are some of the various findings. One of the classic studies was by Gillette and Conway in 1960 in which they differentiated the above two from a normal scar.[48] They tested proliferation of epithelial cells, rate of outgrowth of fibrocytes, mucin production, and histologic sections. Their laboratory findings agreed with their clinical judgement in 85% of the cases. The fibroblasts developed last, at 6-10 days, while the hypertrophic scar developed at 2-3 days with the normal scar falling in between the two. They also found that the clot did not liquify until last in the keloid, with the hypertrophic scar being first and the scar in between. Different cell types were identified: Normal, which are similar to fetal fibroblasts; type I, which have spindle-shaped fibroblasts that migrate into the plasma matrix easily containing numerous mitochondria; and type II, which are large, less mobile, and epitheloid in shape. Type I cells predominate in keloids and hypertrophic scars, and Type II are only present in keloids. The normal cells were less evident in the keloid and hypertrophic scars. Mucin production was present only in keloids and overgrowth of epithelial cells was present only in hypertrophic scars.

In another study by Blackburn in 1966, he used four categories for classification. In a hematoxylin and eosin stain, the collagen fibers were broad and glossy and mucin was present in keloids, but absent in hypertrophic scars. Also, a foreign body reaction and fibroblast were frequently absent in keloids while more abundant in hypertrophic scars. Blackburn felt it important to differentiate the two so that he could evaluate reccurrences and predict better results for surgery. He found 60% of keloids returned, while only 10% of the hypertrophic scars recurred.

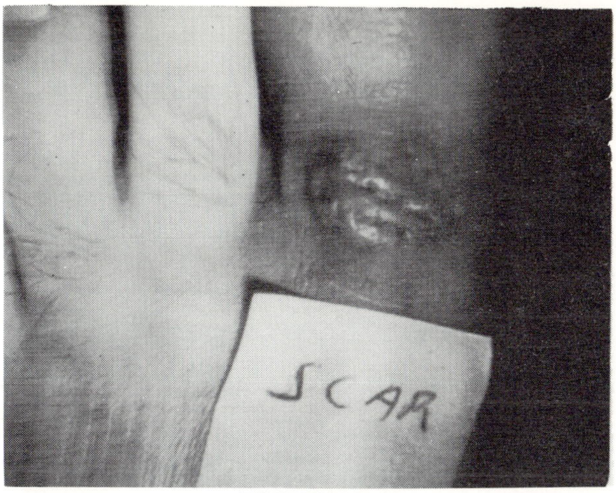

FIGURE 5-39

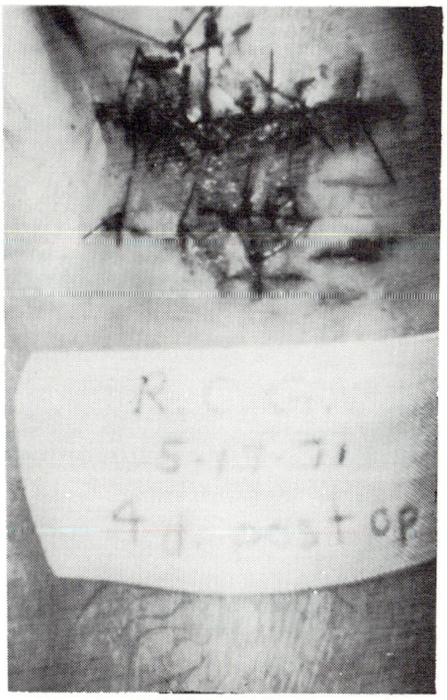

FIGURE 5-40

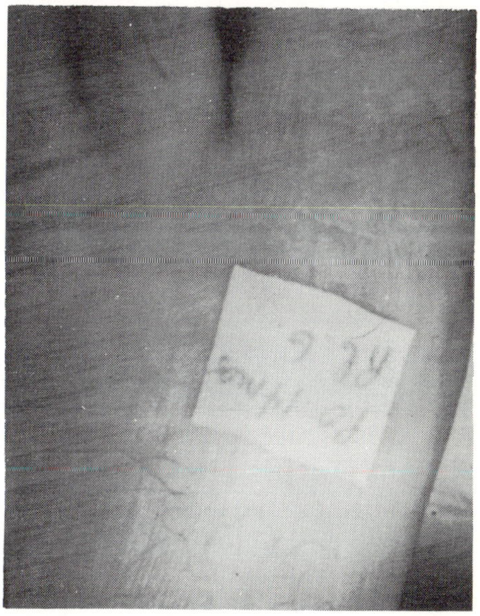

FIGURE 5-41

FIGURES 5-39, 5-40 & 5-41

Hypertrophic Scar: Irregular hypertrophic scar closely resembling a keloid clinically. Surgical excision was performed utilizing multiple skin releases. Fourteen months post-operative there was minimal to no scar.

Peacock believes that all attempts to differentiate the two histiologically, morphologically, or by any other biological or behavorial methods have been unconvincing.[101] He feels that there really is no difference except in the amount of collagen production. The similarities between the two included solubility of the collagen, increase in the proportion between mucopolysaccharides to collagen, lack of organization of fibers and small fiber bundles.

Treatment

There have been quite a number of different means in treating the hypertrophic scars and keloids. This probably infers that there is no best method. Surgery, radiotherapy, and intralesional steroids have been the treatments most often advocated. Some of the methods consisted of enzymes and bile from an Indian turtle, extract from a hog's salivary gland, fibrinolysin, pepsin, hydrochloric acid, hyaluronidase, heparin, Vitamins B^2, C, and E, antimetabolites, nitrogen mustard, thiotepa, chemicals such as formalin and creosote, liquid nitrogen, and injections of hormones. Others included repeated peeling of the scar with the use of a cold quartz lamp, using an electrostatic brush, and ultrasound.[24,36,122,127]

Steroid Treatment

In 1951, Conway and Stark were the first to use steroids in the treatment of scars.[22] They injected adrenocorticotrophic hormone into keloids after excision and achieved some subjective relief of pain and pruritis, but with no improvement of the lesion in three out of the four patients. In other patients, the corticotropin was combined with hyaluronidase and injected directly into the keloids. The hyaluronidase was used to spread the corticotropin. Cortisone has an anti-permeability effect which acts on the connective tissue, synovial fluid, and hyaluronic acid, a ground substance of the skin which binds water in the interstitial spaces, holding the cells together. One of the cases they treated was following a surgical treatment for syndactylism of the toes. The first, second, and third toes of the right foot became fused into a reddened elevated scar. They excised the area and covered it with a split thickenss skin graft. They then gave 60 mg of corticotropin daily for two days, reducing the dosage to 40 mg for the next 20 days. On a follow-up of 8 months, a scar formed at the junction of the graft with the normal skin, but no new keloid developed.

Baker felt that one of the reasons for attempting to use steroids was to decrease the size of the dermis.[6] It caused a complete stoppage in the growth of granulation tissue. The fibroblasts did not proliferate and there were few outgrowths of the endothelial buds from the blood vessels. Also, the fibroblasts present in the connective tissue did not mature. Then, in 1951, Cornman was able to demonstrate that deoxycorticosterone changed the shape and size of the fibroblasts.[25] It was not until 1963, when Murray reported improvement in keloids due to injection of triamcinolone acetate, that definite improvements in the treatment were begun.[97] In this initial study, he excised the scar by surgery first, then deposited Kenalog (Squibb) at the surgical site. He stated that the keloid was delayed in forming until six months, when it redeveloped. His mistake was that he used only one injection. He then advocated a combined method of treatment by using excision, followed by injection of Kenalog and topical applications of Kenalog with irradiation of 800r in divided doses. He found that the topical Kenalog resulted in a flatter and broader scar. In 1965, Maguire injected 25 mg/ml of Kenalog ranging from 35-715 mg in 56 cases. 51 became soft and flat, 32 disappeared, and in 5, there was no difference.[87]

In 1966, Griffith recommended injection of Kenalog into the wound area after totally excising the keloid.[51] Even greater results and less recurrence were obtained by giving additional injections post-operatively. He was able to follow up his patients and reported in 1970 that out of 103 patients, 90% were effectively reduced or eliminated by injections alone.[52] In five of the patients, the keloid returned but was re-treated with Kenalog causing the lesion to flatten out. One disadvantage that he did find when combining intralesional injections with excision was subcutaneous atrophy and spreading of the scar.

Ketchum also produced good results while using intralesional injections of Kenalog.[74,75] He stated the injection of Kenalog intralesionally produced relief of paresthesia and regression in both hypertrophic scars and keloids in about 95% of 195 treated. Within three to five days the pruritis and paresthesia decreased and within three weeks time a moderate to marked reduction in the amount of scar tissue was noticed. He found the best results are obtained if excision was combined with the injection and related his own formula to the age and size of the lesions. At first he experienced results causing atrophy and depigmentation. He found that these adverse reactions could be avoided by injecting only into the scar and not into normal tissue beneath or adjacent to the scar. Better responses were also found to occur in younger patients and in scars that were newly formed.

Injection of triamcinalone acetonide, or Aristocort (Lederle) seems to produce the same results. It is uncommon to get a local reaction and systemic reactions are rare. Kenalog is well tolerated, has a low toxicity and is an effective anti-inflammatory agent. One should inject with care those with tuberculosis, chronic and acute infection and osteoporosis. The most adverse reaction is atrophy and depigmentation which usually disappears with time. Other local reactions may be pain, discomfort, hemorrhage, infection, hypersensitivity, and wound dehiscence. One may reduce complications by injecting directly into the lesion and not the surrounding tissue, using sterile techniques, and varying the solubility of the steroids in multiple injections.

Steroids have been tried orally, intramuscularly, local injections, or a combination of all. Orally, cortisone and hydrocortisone tend to cause salt and water retention and hypertension, and is therefore useful when hydration is recommended. Prednisone and prednisolone cause less salt and water retention, but more potassium depletion. Systemic steroids are not indicated in the management of this localized lesion.

Steroids inhibit sulfuration of mucopolysaccharide in ground substance. The local injections of steroid are supposed to cause the collagen to dissolve. This is probably due to inhibition of protein synthesis, acting as a depolymerising agent making scars more susceptible to tissue collagenoses. The protocol as to how much and how often varies with the type, age, and the doctor treating the lesion. Below are some of the regimes:

1. Inject 0.5 to 1.0 ml of triamcinolone acetate weekly, biweekly, as often as necessary, or until no benefits are seen.[119]
2. A 50-50 mixture of Xylocaine with Kenalog injected every two weeks until regression.

When injecting in the beginning, a great deal of resistance may be encountered. The use of a small gauge syringe relieves the back pressure. It is recommended that the area be blocked locally with 1% lidocaine hydrochloride, and a 25 gauge needle be used. Or, one may use a Dermojet to introduce the corticosteroid. Multiple injections may be given 0.5 cm apart, but the patient will probably experience pain due to stretching and pressure. With each injection, the lesion will become softer. The older the scar, the longer the treatment.

Topical steroids are also used, in fact, some recommend using this method before attempting surgery, or using it as an adjunct.[140] Fluocinolone acetonide has been shown to be one of the most potent anti-inflammatory and fibroblastic suppressing steroids tested to date. The 0.2% cream, Synalar HP (Syntex), is used twice per day and hopefully it will cause the excess scar to flatten.

Steroids may be used in conjunction with irradiation. It has been reported that it may result in a finer scar. Radium and X-ray either alone, or in conjunction with excision, was the treatment of choice until the usage of intralesional injection of steroids. Steroids have been recommended over irradiation because of the possible side effects following X-ray therapy. One should be extremely careful in irradiation of children as damage may be done to the epiphysis. Other complications of the skin may be hypo- or hyperpigmentation, radiodermatitis, and radionecrosis. But, irradiation, properly given, is an effective treatment for both keloids and hypertrophic scars. The young, developing, vascular buds in a new wound are radiosensitive and therefore can be retarded.

The irradiation limits the proliferation of the young fibroblasts by decreasing the amount of collagen being produced. Irradiation works best if started within 3 days after excision or re-excision of the scar. If the keloid or hypertrophic scar is old and thickened, irradiation will not reduce the size of the lesion, but will help the itching and burning symptoms.

There has been no agreement as to the proper dosage of irradiation for the treatment of the scars. It is generally agreed that excision should be done before irradiation. However, both superficial and Grenz ray therapy have been utilized.

Surgery and Precautions

Excision of a keloid is usually employed with other means of treatment. All skin incisions produce permanent scars, but a good surgeon tries to minimize the scar formation and make it as inconspicuous as possible. To achieve this, good sound surgical procedure should be followed. There are many factors which affect wound healing and should be thought of by the surgeon before surgery. The patient's nutrition and health are very important. A patient may not heal as well if he has just recovered from any systematic illnesses, such as an infection or hepatitis, or if he has just been on a diet and lost a great deal of weight. Chronic drug or alcohol use impair the healing procedure. An anabolic state should exist with proper protein intake and good health.

Incisions are best located in "hidden areas," such as hair bearing areas, skin lines of tension, wrinkle and contour lines. Wrinkle lines occur in the skin at right angles to the axis of contraction of underlying muscle. Pinching the skin may reveal the natural wrinkle lines when muscle contraction is not helpful. Contour lines occur on the skin surface between different skin textures or different body structures. Lines of Langer are not always a good reference, as his work was performed on cadavers. Incisions should be vertical to the skin so that the blood supply will be disturbed as little as possible. Asepsis, meticulous hemostasis, careful wound apposition with slight eversion and avoidance of tension of the skin reduces wound fibroplasia. Aggressive control of infected wounds, extraction of foreign bodies, immobilization of the wound by splinting, pressure dressings, or plaster casts all improve the chances of a finer scar. Dressings should support the suture line to prevent tension. Bandages can range from the normal 2x2 and kling to a more elaborate type such as advocated by two Japanese surgeons.[43] They used self-adhering poly-urethane foam, which permits passage of air, sweat, and secretions, but is not irritating. An elastic bandage is placed over this and left in place until healing is mature, which may be weeks or months. This is judged by noticing the fading of the redness. This treatment was only useful in hypertrophic scars and not keloids, which was their method in differentiating the two.

The excising of a keloid with no other treatment usually results in the keloid returning larger than the original size. This is especially true when you resect normal tissue along with the scar causing an increase in wound tension. When excising a scar, some advocate removing the entire lesion, while others leave a small amount of the lesion in the wound. The reason partial excision may work is that the periphery may act as a splint, preventing retraction of the wound edges.[101] When excising a scar, the tension surrounding the wound must be relieved, otherwise, no matter what type of suture or steroid you use, the scar tissue will return. L-shaped Z-plasties, or split thickness skin grafts (STSG), may be used to relieve skin tension. If the area to be excised is large, a split thickness skin graft would most likely have to be used. If a STSG is required, use a thin take of 8/1000 to 10/1000 ins., or a keloid may occur in the donor site. Also, take a graft where continued pressure can be applied. If the lesion can be removed without leaving too much tension, primary closure is attempted, using 4-0 plain catgut subcutaneously, continuous subcuticular sutures of stainless steel wire, 32 gauge, and skin closure with 4-0 nylon.

Prognosis

Keloids require greater care in treatment and are more highly resistant to both conservative and surgical management than hypertrophic scars.

6. CUTANEOUS MUCOUS CYSTS (MYXOID CYSTS)

Clinical Consideration

Cutaneous mucous cysts are small, single or multiple, soft, transluscent-to-reddish lesions over the terminal interphalangeal joints of the finger, and less commonly the toes. They contain a clear, viscid to gray, jelly-like material and commonly undergo spontaneous or traumatic rupture, but nearly always regenerate within 2 to 4 weeks.[147] These growths may cause longitudinal grooving or nail dystrophy when the cysts overlie the proximal nail fold (matrix) area. Cutaneous mucous cysts are more commonly found in females, usually between the ages of 40 and 65.[16] A sac or swelling may also be seen proximal to the cyst, with a duct appearance leading from the joint to the cyst.

Review of the Literature

Hyde first described 43 cases of these multiple cysts of the digits, of which five cases were on the toes, in 1893.[66] He believed

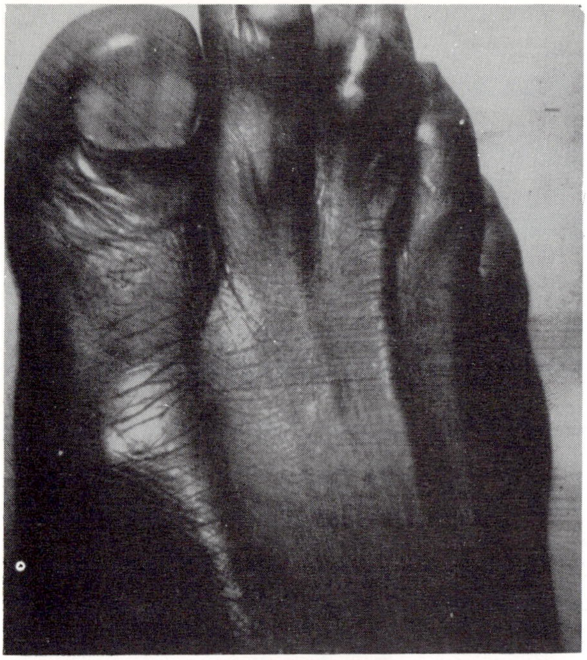

FIGURE 5-42

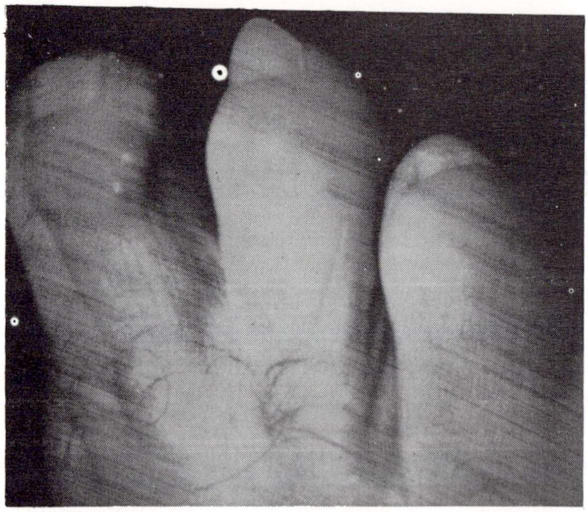

FIGURE 5-43

Cutaneous Mucous Cysts: These lesions are usually asymptomatic. Involvement of the nail often results in dystrophic changes. (Courtesy of Jeff Yale, D.P.M., Ansonia, Conn.)

they were projections of synovial fluid into the skin. In his early editions, Lever classified mucous cysts as myxomas, which are very rare in the skin and are usually subungual.[83] Recent studies have concluded that these subepidermal cysts are due to a connective tissue defect in which excessive fibroblasts in the corium secrete hyaluronic acid which decreases collagen formation, and the subsequent spaces fill with mucin.[71,83]

Histopathology

Early in their course, cutaneous mucous cysts have the same microscopic appearance as cutaneous myxoma.[83] Later, there is an intradermal, non-encapsulated collection of connective tissue mucin with fibroblastic infiltration. Hyaluronic acid is detected on chemical study.[71]

Differential Diagnosis

Differential diagnosis is quite difficult. It includes epidermoid cyst, fibroma, ganglionic cyst, Heberden's node, xanthoma, verruca vulgaris, heloma, and vesicles or bulla of mycotic origin.[147]

Prognosis

Although benign, these cysts are persistent, and recurrence is the rule following most modes of therapy.

Treatment

Many authors suggest surgical excision, but warn about recurrences.[16,147] Intralesional injection of steroid preparations (usually triamcinolone) have yielded varied results[71] [147] Radiation therapy has yielded good results by those trained to administer it.[23,68]

7. DERMATOFIBROSARCOMA PROTUBERANS

Definition

Dermatofibrosarcoma protuberans is a fibrosarcoma of the skin, usually of low grade malignancy, but rarely metastasize. The term "dermatofibrosarcoma protuberans" is generally not the correct terminology since these neoplasms usually do not metastasize.

Histology

The earliest description of this disease was by Taylor, in 1890, however, it was Darier and Ferrance, in 1924, who described the unusual progressive recurring tumor of the skin.[31] A year later Hoffman reported several similar cases and coined the term "dermatofibrosarcoma protuberans."[60]

Incidence

Dermatofibrosarcoma protuberans occurs most often in young and middle aged adults.[62 100] Pack found 39 cases (5.4%) of DFSP out of 717 cases of malignant tumors of the soft tissues.[100] Burkhardt, et al, in a series of 56 cases, found the mean age of onset at 28 years; in two-thirds of the patients, the tumor occurred during the first four decades of life.[19] Holms states that the distribution in the sexes is equal, whereas in Burkhardt's study, the tumor occurred in males in 57% of the cases.[19 62] Pack reports 61.5% occurrence in males. This tumor has rarely been reported on the foot.

Etiology

The etiology of dermatofibrosarcoma protuberans is unknown, and, according to Holm, there are no predisposing factors related to its development.

Clinical Picture

The most common sites of dermatofibrosarcoma protuberans are the abdomen, back, groin, thigh, and chest, although it has been described on every part of the cutaneous surface, except the palms and soles.[62,100] Dermatofibrosarcoma protuberans usually starts as one or several small, hard, reddish, bluish or brownish nodules which may coalesce to form one or several keloid-like plaques. From these plaques, protruding fibrous tumors develop. These may be sessile or pedunculated, and are markedly protuberant, sometimes reaching the size of a fist, and are of irregular contour. A mushroom-like lobulation may form. The tumor is generally hard and painless. Eventually, ulceration may occur. The tumor is locally invasive, but metastases are exceedingly uncommon.[62,100] In Burkhardt's study, 7 of the 56 cases involved the lower extremity (12.5%) with 5 of these on the thigh and 2 on the leg. Kulchar states they may also occur on the foot.[81]

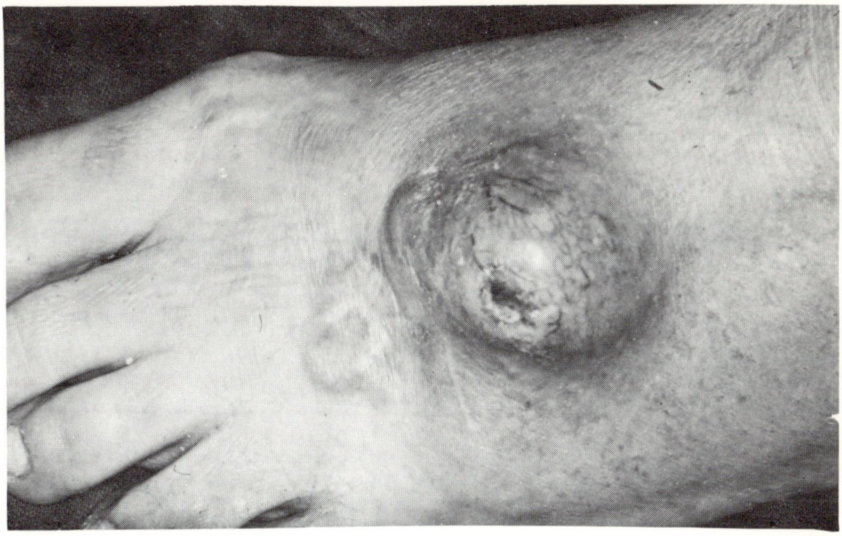

FIGURE 5-44

Large dermatofibrosarcoma protuberance, dorsal surface of the foot. (Courtesy of the Armed Forces Institute of Pathology.)

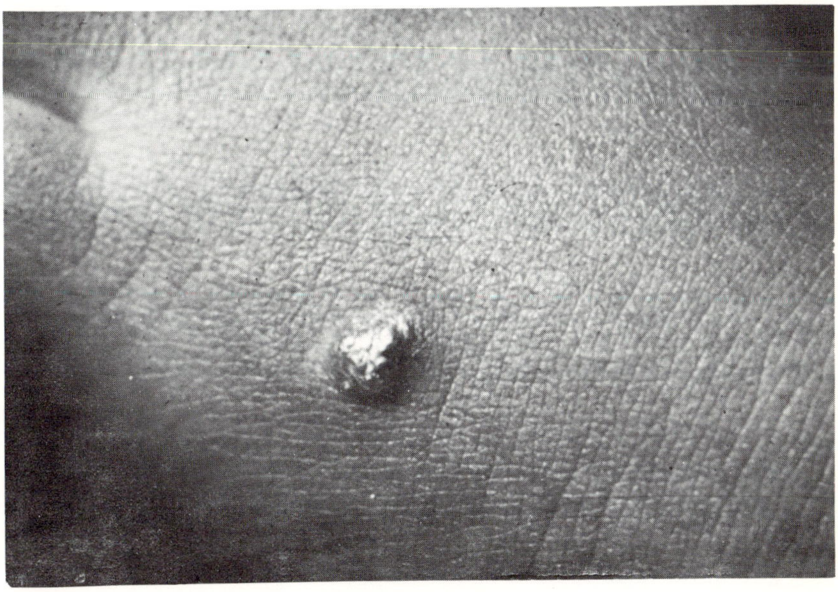

FIGURE 5-45

Dermatofibrosarcoma protuberance, dorsal lateral surface of the foot. (Courtesy of the Armed Forces Institute of Pathology.)

The diagnosis of dermatofibrosarcoma must be made on a combination of clinical evidence and histologic features. The tumor is fixed to both the surrounding skin and to the subcutaneous fat and fascia. At times, regression, and even involution, may take place spontaneously, but fatal metastases have been reported.[62 81]

Pathology

The tumor is considered to be intermediate in position between fibroma and sarcoma and is frequently mistaken by the pathologist for neurofibroma or neurogenic sarcoma. It may be confused with fibrosarcoma. The tumors develop in the cutis as small nodules that increase in size and may invade the underlying adipose tissue and fascia at the same time as the tumor becomes more and more protuberant.

Treatment

The base of dermatofibrosarcoma protuberans tends toward lateral occult spread. This accounts for approximately 20% recurrence rate following local excision.[102] Wide excision is the treatment of choice; follow-up must be continued for years because recurrences may appear late. These tumors have a great tendency to be infiltrative to other areas of the body tissues. Many times skin grafting is necessary to close the defect. If the dermatofibrosarcoma infiltrates the fascia surrounding the muscle, the involved muscle layer should be excised. It is a highly radio-resistant tumor.[62 102]

Prognosis

This tumor carries an excellent prognosis after adequate wide excision even though the local recurrence rate is high and despite the histologic similarity to fibrosarcoma.[19 102]

HEMANGIOMA

Definition

Vascular tumors of the pedal skin are not uncommon. This monograph series will only consist of the vascular lesions as they may limit themselves to the skin. Vascular tumors such as pyogenic granuloma, Kaposi's sarcoma, and cavernous hemangiomas will be deleted from this monograph series.

Hemangiomas are benign tumors which are usually derived or composed of epithelial cells and are lined with vascular spaces. The majority of these lesions as classified on the pedal skin are primarily spoken of as capillary hemangiomas.

1. *Capillary hemangiomas (strawberry)* – are the most common of all the hemangiomas occuring in the skin and mucous membrane. Synonyms for capillary hemangioma are nevus vasculosis, strawberry hemangioma.

2. *Spider Hemangioma (nevus araneus)* - usually appears as a very small central growth ranging in size from less than a millimeter to two millimeters in size. Its surrounding body may appear as a sunburst or a spider.

3. *Port-wine stain (nevus flammeus)* These are superficial hemangiomas which are usually first noticed at birth and continue to develop as the individual grows. It appears as a reddish to

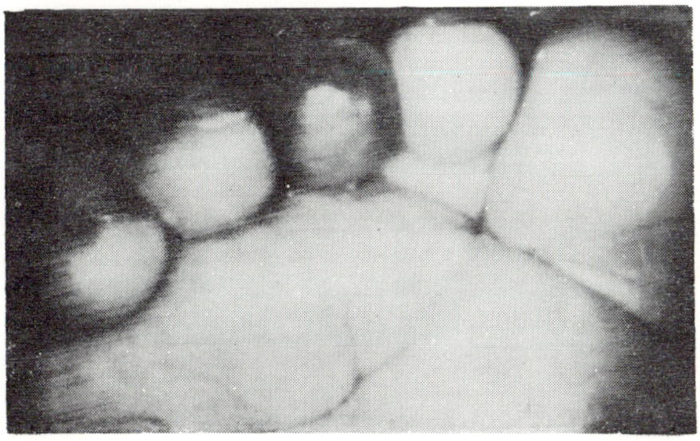

FIGURE 5-46

Strawberry Hemangioma: Strawberry hemangioma of the middle digit in an infant.

purple flat superficial mass and/or coloring of the skin. The port-wine stain unfortunately, has a tendency to remain throughout life, and does produce a cosmetic deformity particulary when it involes the face, head, and neck areas. Fortunately, its involvement on the pedal extremities is quite uncommon, and usually has no bearing on one's pedal health. Histologically, these lesions usually present themselves with thin-walled capillary cavernous type vessels, loosely arranged within the dermal layers of the skin. They may also in certain instances, show similar patterns to cavernous hemangiomas.

Clinical Picture

Capillary hemangioma is perhaps the most common tumor in association with infancy and childhood. The majority of thes(hemangiomas are usually associated with the superficial areas o the skin. They are usually first noted shortly after birth, oı within the first month after birth. Fitzwilliam sited 649 cases and over 83% of the hemangiomas were first noted at birth.[138] Ap-

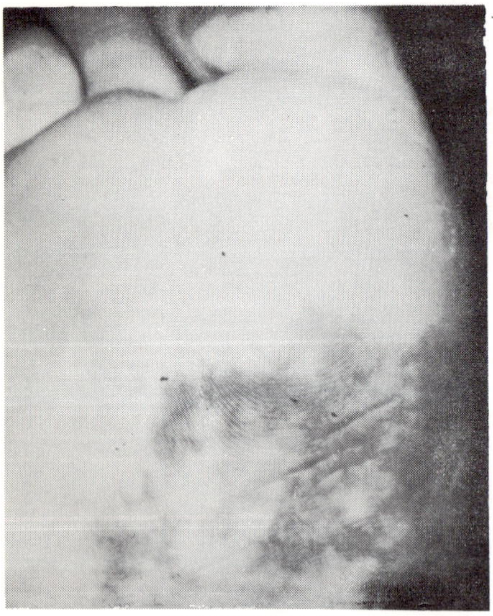

FIGURE 5-47

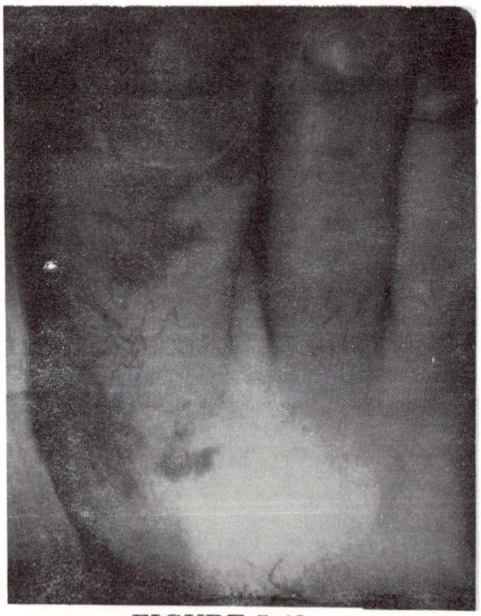

FIGURE 5-48

Port Wine Stain Hemangioma: Port wine stain of the plantar surface of the foot, and the dorsal surface, hallux toe. Lesions are asymptomatic and require no treatment.

pearance on the head and neck comprise the greatest majority of cases occuring during infancy. Hemangiomas on the foot during infancy are quite uncommon. Fortunately, the majority of the superficial hemangiomas do have a tendency to convolute and disappear. Capillary hemangiomas vary greatly in size and may extend into the subcutaneous tissues. Their clinical appearance usually presents a smooth surface, however, it may be irregular and slightly elevated. The superficial lesions are usually bright red in color (strawberry), but those lesions which may have deeper components have a tendency to be darker in color (port-wine). The lesions are often compressible, but seldom completely blanch when pressure is applied. These lesions may have a tendency to grow rapidly after birth. There are multiple factors which stimulate growth of vascular tumors, yet none of them are clearly understood. Injury to certain areas may contribute or stimulate growth rate in vascular lesions, and are often associated with clinical symptoms. Fortunately, the majority of these lesions do have a tendency to disappear, usually by the age of three. If the lesions continue to grow, these lesions may possibly develop to cavernous forms of hemangiomas, and in some instances may even suggest the possibility of a malignancy.

Diagnosis

The diagnosis is usually easily made and is seldom a problem. Superficial capillary types of hemangiomas that limit themselves to the dermal areas of the skin are usually no problem to diagnose. Difficulty, however, does arise when these lesions continue to grow and involve deeper tissue areas.

Differential Diagnosis

Fortunately, the diagnosis of these skin hemangiomas are quite easily made. It should be pointed out, however, that the spider hemangiomas may be associated with Rendu Oslars Weber's Disease, liver disease, A vitaminosis, and deficiency in Vitamin B. Port-wine stains, on the other hand, may be associated with Sturge-Weber syndrome and Klipple-Trenaunay syndrome.

Treatment

Many therapies have been described in the literature, whether it be cryotherapy, injection therapy, radiation, or various forms of surgical treatment. Capillary hemangiomas most often should be left alone, and, usually after a period of a few years, often involute and spontaneously disappear. Spider hemangioma, on the other hand, is usually simply and successfully treated by electrocautery. The port-wine stain, unfortunately, does not respond well to any form of therapy. It usually persists through the individual's life. Overzealous treatment often results in complications, for example: sclerosing therapy may develop embolism, allergy or scarring of the skin by ulceration. Radiation therapy, if utilized in children, may injure various growth centers involving the bones of the foot, creating even greater deformity than the skin lesion itself.

Prognosis

Capillary hemangioma and spider hemangioma seldom present a problem, and often disappear spontaneously or by simple treatment. The port-wine stain persists throughout life.

BIBLIOGRAPHY

1. Allen, A. C.: *The Skin,* ed. 2, Grune & Stratton, New York, 1967.
2. Allen, P. W.: Recurring digital fibrous tumors of childhood, *Pathology,* 4:215-223, 1972.
3. Arner, O., et al: Mucous cysts of the fingers. *Acta. Chir. Scand.,* **111**:314-321, 1956.
4. Arnold, H. L., et al, Keloids: etiology and management by excision and intensive prophylactic radiation, *Arch. Derm.,* **80**:772, 1959.
5. Asboe, Hansen G., et al: Treatment of keloids with topical injections of hydrocortisone acetate. *Arch. Derm.,* **73**:162, 1965.
6. Baker, B., et al: Interference with wound healing by local action of adrenocortical steroids. *Endocrinology,* **46**:544, 1950.
7. Banfield, W., et al: Acetic acid-soluble collagen in human scars. *Surg. Gynec. & Obstet.,* **109**:367, 1959.
8. Baruch, K.: Injection method treatment of porokeratosis. *J. Podiatric Educ.,* **3**:1, 1972.
9. Belisario, J.: The Treatment of Keloids. *Acta. Dermat. Venerol.* **37**:165, 1957.
10. Berlin, S. J.: *Hemangiomas of the Foot: Report of four cases and Review of the Literature.* Volume 60, 1970, page 63.
11. Berlin, S. J.: Epidermal inclusion cyst of the foot: Report of three cases. *JAPA,* **61**:55-58, 1971.
12. Berliner, D. C.: Decreased scar formation with topical corticosteriod treatments. *Surgery,* **61**:619, 1967.
13. Bernstein, H.: Treatment of keloids by steroids with biochemical tests for diagnosis and prognosis. *Angiology,* **15**:253, 1964.
14. Binkley, G. W.: Dermatofibrosarcoma protuberans: Report of six cases. *Arch. Derm. and Syph.,* **40**:589, 1939.

15. Blackburn, W. R., et al: Histiologic basis of keloid and hypertrophic scar differentation. *Arch. Path.*, **82**:65, 1966.
16. Bourns, H. K. and Sanerkin, N. G.: Mucoid lesions of the fingers and toes. *Brit. J. Surg.*, **60**:860, 1963.
17. Brown, J., et al: Preliminary studies on the effect of patterns in the treatment of keloids. *Radiology*, **80**:298, 1963.
18. Brown, J. B. and Fryer, M. P.: Hemangiomas: Role of plastic surgery in early treatment for prevention of deformities and in repair of late lesions and defects. *Plast. Reconstr. Surg.*, **11**:197, 1953.
19. Burkhardt, B. R., et al: Dermatofibrosarcoma protuberans: Study of fifty-six cases. *Am. J. Surg.*, **111**:638, 1966.
20. Busch, J.: *Dermatol. Z.*, 11, 1931 (cited in Skeer, J.: Adenoma Sebaceum Pringle), von Recklinghausen's disease, subungual fibromatosis associated with epilepsy or tuberous sclerosis, a symptom complex. *Urol. Cutan. Rev.*, **42**:110, 1938.
21. Campbell, R. J.: Epidermal inclusion cyst of foot with foreign body reaction. *JAPA*, **55**:210-211, 1965.
22. Conway, H., et al: Corticotropin (ACTH) in treatment of keloids. *Arch. of Surgery*, **64**:47, 1952.
23. Conway, H., Hugo, N. E., and Tulenko, J. F.: *Surgery of Tumors of the Skin*, 2nd ed., Thomas, Springifeld, Ill., 1966.
24. Cornbleet, T.: Treatment of Keloids with Hyaluronidose. *JAMA*, **154**:1161, 1954.
25. Cornman, I.: Selective damage to fibroblasts by deoxycorticosterone in cultures. *Science*, **113**:37, 1951.
26. Cosman, B.: Correlation of keloid recurrence with completeness of local excision. *Plast. Reconstr. Surg.*, **50**:163, 1972.
27. Cosman, B., et al: The Surgical Treatment of Keloids. *Plast. Reconstr. Surg.*, **27**:335, 1961.
28. Costello, M. and Gibbs, R.: *The Palms and Soles in Medicine*. Springfield, Ill., 1967, C. Thomas.
29. Craig, R. D., et al: Early post-operative irradication in the treatment of keloid scars. *Brit. J. Plast. Surg.*, **18**:369, 1965.
30. Crockett, D.: Regional keloid susceptability. *Brit. J. Plast. Surg.*, **17**:245, 1964.
31. Darier, J., et al: Dermatofibromes progressibs et recidivants. *Ann. de Dermat. and Syph.*, **5**:545, 1924.
32. Dave. V. K.: Keloid, *Physiotherapy*, **56**:97, 1970.
33. Deigert, F. A.: Keloids: Reassessment of irradiation therapy. *Rocky Mt. Med. J.*, **70**:35, 1973.
34. Dix. R.: Epidermoid cyst following osteotrypsy. *JAPA*, **62**:114, 1972.
35. Dribbon, B.: The utilization of an alcohol-local anesthetic solution in the treatment of the plugged duct cyst. *JAPA*, **61**:203, 1971.
36. Du Vries, H.: *Surgery of The Foot*. St. Louis, 1965, C. V. Mosby, Co.
37. Edgertown, M.: Use of Vitamin E in the treatment of keloids. *Plast. Reconstr. Surg.*, **8**:224, 1951.
38. Evans, R. W.: *Histiologic Appearance of Tumors*. Baltimore., Williams & Wilkins, 1966.
39. Feinstein, M.: Foot pathology associated with tuberous sclerosis and neurofibromatosis. *JAPA*, **9**:336-362, 1972.
40. Fine, H. L.: Keloids containing hair and sebaceous glands. *Arch. Derm.*, **96**:185, 1967.

41. Fitzpatrick, et al: *Dermatology in General Medicine*. McGraw-Hill, Inc., 1971.
42. Freeman, R. G., Knox, J. M., and Spiller, W. F.: Eccrine poroma. *Am. J. Clin. Path.*, **36**:444-450, 1961.
43. Fujimori, R., et al: Sponge fixation method for treatment of early scars. *Plast. Reconstr. Surg.*, **42**:322, 1968.
44. Galenski, A.: Recurrent digital fibroma of childhood. *JAMA,* **62**:114, 1972.
45. Gates, O., et al: Tumors of sweat glands. *Am. J. Path.*, **19**:591-631, 1943.
46. German, A. I.: Eccrine proma. Review of the literature and case report. *Arch. Derm.*, **89**:382-384, 1964.
47. Gibbs, R. C.: Eccrine poroma. *JAPA,* **58**:298-300, 1968.
48. Gillette, R. and Conway, H.: A differential diagnosis of keloids and hypertrophic scars by tissue culture techniques with notes on therapy of keloids by surgical excision and decadron. *Plast. Reconstr. Surg.,* **25**:117, 1960.
49. Goldman, L.: Reaction following intralesional and sublesional injection of corticosteroids. *JAMA,* **182**:613, 1962.
50. Goldner, R.: Eccrine poromatosis. *Arch. Derm.,* **101**:606, 1970.
50A. Greev, K. E.: Epidermal inclusion cyst of the sole. *Arch Derm.*, Feb. 1974.
51. Griffith, B.: Treatment of keloids with triamcinolone acetonide. *Plast. Reconstr. Surg.,* **38**:202, 1966.
52. Griffith, B., et al: Follow-up study on the treatment of keloids with triamcinolone acetonide. *Plast. Reconstr. Surg.,* **46**:145, 1970.
53. Griswold, T.: Effects of adrenal cortical preparations on scar hypertrophy. *Plast. Reconstr. Surg.*, **133**:454, 1954.
54. Gross, F.: Sclerosing hemangiomas — their relationship to dermatofibroma, histiocytoma, xanthoma and to certain pigmented lesions of the skin. *Am. J. Path.,* **9**:533, 1943.
55. Gross, R. E.: Recurring myxomatous cutaneous cysts of the fingers and toes. *Surg. Gynec. & Obst.,* **65**:289, 1937.
56. Gross, S.: Sebaceous cysts. *JAMA,* **152**:813, 1953.
57. Grunnet, N., et al: Recurring digital fibrous tumor of childhood. *Acta. Pathol., Microbiol. Scand.,* **81**:167, 1973.
58. Hare, P. J.: Eccrine poroma of the sole. *Proc. Royal Soc. Med.,* **54**:697, 1961.
59. Heierli, E.: Porokeratosis of mantoux. *Dermatologica,* **119**:309, 1959.
60. Hoffman, E.: Uber das Knollentreibende Fibrosarkom der Haut (Dermatofibrosarkoma Protuberans). *Derm. Ztschr.* **43**:1, 1925.
61. Hogan, V. M.: Cutaneous scars and cosmetic surgery. *Surg. Clin. N. Amer.,* **51**:491, 1971.
62. Holm, J.: Dermatofibrosarcoma protuberans. Report of a case with review of the literature. *Acta. Chir. Scand.,* **134**:303, 1968.
63. Hoopes, J. E., et al: Enzyme activities in hypertrophic scars and keloids. *Plast. Reconstr. Surg.,* **47**:137, 1971.
64. Horton, C.: Malignant changes in keloids. *Plast. Reconstr. Surg.,* **12**:86, 1953.
65. Hunter, G. A. and Donald, G. T.: Eccrine proma: A review of the literature and discussion of six personal cases. *Austr. J. Derm.,* **6**:58, 1961.
66. Hyde, J. N.: *Practical Treatise on Diseases of Skin.* Hency C. Lea's Son & Co., Phila., 1883, p. 42.
67. Hyman, A. B. and Brownstein, M. H.: Eccrine poroma. *Dermatologica,* **138**:29-38, 1969.

68. Issacson, N. H. and McCarty, D.: Recurring myxomatous cutaneous cyst. *Surgery,* **35**:621, 1954.
69. Jao, J., et al: Lymphangiomyoma and tuberous sclerosis. *Cancer,* May, 1972.
70. Johnson, F.: Now More Procedure for the Assay of H^3 or C^{14} Labelled Hydroxyprolene. *Anal. Biochem.,* **15**:77, 1966.
71. Johnson, W. C., et al: Cutaneous myxoid cyst. *JAMA,* **191**:15, 1965.
72. Juna K., et al: Modified procedure for the assay of H^3 or C^{14} labelled hydroxyprolene. *Anal. Biochem.,* **15**:77, 1966.
73. Kaufmann: Histiocytic tumors (fibrous xanthoma and histiocytoma) in children. *Cancer,* **14**:469, 1961.
74. Ketchum, L. D., et al: Treatment of hypertrophic scars, keloid and scar contracture by triamcinolone acetonide. *Plast. Reconstr. Surg.,* **38**:209, 1966.
75. Ketchum, L. D., et al: Follow-up on treatment of hypertrophic scars and keloids with triamcinolone. *Plast. Reconstr. Surg.* **48**:256, 1971.
76. King, G. D., et al: Keloid scars. *Surg. Clin. of N. Amer.,* **50**:595, 1970.
77. Kitlowski, E.: Treatment of keloids and keloidal scars. *Plast. Reconstr. Surg.,* **12**:383, 1953.
78. Kligman, A. M.: The myth of the sebaceous cyst. *Arch. Derm.,* **89**:253, 1964.
79. Koonin, A. J.: Etiology of keloids. *S. Afr. Med. J.,* **38**:913, 1964.
80. Kothe: Berliner Thieraerztliche Wochenschrift. 1903.
81. Kulchar, G. V.: Benign and malignant tumors of the foot. *JAMA,* **124**:761, 1944.
82. Lampel I. and Latourette, H. B.: Management of cavernous hemangiomas in infants. *Pediat. Clin. N. Amer.,* **6**:511, 1959.
83. Lever, W. F.: *Histopathology of the Skin,* Lippincott, Phila., 1971, 4th ed. p. 573.
84. Longacre, J., et al: Relationship of ultrastructure of collagen to scar formation and its surgical management. *Brit. J. Plast. Surg.,* **21**:49, 1968.
85. Love, W. R. and Montgomery, H.: Epithelial cysts. *Arch. Derm. & Syph.,* **47**:185, 1943.
86. Maclin, T. B.: Post-traumatic epidermal inclusion cysts; a case report. *JAPA,* **55**:209, 1965.
87. Maguire, H.: Treatment of keloids with triamcinolone acetonide injected intralesionally. *JAMA,* **192**:325, 1965.
88. Margilith, A. M. and Museles, M.: Current concepts in diagnosis and management of congenital cutaneous hemangiomas. *Ped.,* **36**:410, 1965.
89. Margilith, A. M. and Museles, M.: Cutaneous hemangioma in children. *JAMA,* **194**:523, 1965.
90. Marples, M. J.: Ecology of the human skin. Thomas, Springfield, Ill., 1965.
91. McGavran, M. H. and Binnington, B.: Keratinous cysts of the skin. *Arch. Derm.,* **94**:499, 1966.
92. Mehregan, et al: Recurring digital fibrous tumor of childhood. *Arch. Derm.,* September, 1972, p. 106.
93. Mikhail, G. R. and Wertheimer, J.: Porokeratosis. *Arch. Derm.,* **105**:267-296, 1972.
94. Minkowitz, F.: Regression of massive keloid following partial excision and post-operative intralesional administration of triamcinolone. *Brit. J. Plast. Surg.,* **20**:432, 1967.
95. Montgomery, H.: *Dermatopathology,* Vol. 2. Hoeber, N.Y., 1967.

96. Morrell, J. F.: Pilonidal sinus of the sole. *Arch. Derm.*, **75**:269, 1957.
97. Murray, R.: Kenalog and the treatment of hypertrophied scars and keloids in negroes and whites. *Plast. Reconstr. Surg.*, **31**:275, 1963.
98. Niemi, K. M.: Benign fibrohistiocytic tumor of skin. *Acta. Derm. Venereol. Suppl.* **50**(63):1, 1970.
99. Okun, M. R., et al: Eccrine poroma: Report of three cases. *Arch. Derm.*, **88**:561-566, 1963.
100. Pack, G. t.: Liposarcoma: A study of 105 cases. *Surg.*, **36**:687, 1954.
101. Peacock, E. and Van Winkle, W.: *Surgery and Biology of Wound Repair.* W. B. Saunders, Phila., 1970.
102. Pillsbury, D. M., et al: *Dermatology.* W. B. Saunders, Phila., 1956.
103. Pinkus, H., Rogin, J. R., and Goldman, P.: Eccrine poroma. *Arch. Derm.*, **74**:51121, 1956.
104. Pinkus, H.: Porokeratosis. *Arch. Derm.*, **102**:235-236, 1970.
105. Pinkus, H.: Sebaceous cysts are trichilemmal cysts. *Arch. Derm.*, **99**:544, 1969.
106. Psillikes, J.: Water and electrolyte content of normal skin, scars and keloids. *Plast. Reconstr. Surg.*, **47**:272, 1971.
107. Reed, R.: Acral fibrokeratomas. *Arch. Derm.*, **103**:286-297, 1971.
108. Reye, R. D.: Recurring digital fibrous tumors of childhood. *Arch. Path.*, **80**:228-231, 1965.
109. Robbins, S.: *Pathology.* W. B. Saunders, 1967, Phila.
110. Rochese, F.: ACTH and cortisone in the treatment of keloids. *New England J. Med.*, **250**:238, 1954.
111. Rook A., Wilkinson, D. S., and Eibling, F. J. G.: *Textbook of Dermatology.* Davis, Phila., 1968.
112. Rosenberg, A.: A clinical report of atypical dermoid cyst. *JAPA*, **50**:726-728, 1960.
113. Sachatello, C. R. and McSwain, B.: Regression of cutaneous capillary hemangioma. *Amer. J. Surg.*, **116**:113, 1968.
114. Samitz, M. H. and Dana, A. S.: *Cutaneous Lesions of the Lower Extremities.* Lippincott, Phila., 1971.
115. Sanderson, K. V. and Ryan, E. A.: Histochemisty of eccrine poroma. *Birt. J. Derm.*, **75**:86-88, 1963.
116. Saunders, T. S.: Porokeratosis: A disease of the epidermal eccrine sweat duct units. *Arch. Derm.*, **84**:980-988, 1961.
117. Schultze, H. A.: Hair as a penetrating foreign body in the plantar surface of the foot. *Arch. Derm. & Syph.*, **61**:668, 1950.
118. Shapiro, L.: Infantile digital fibromatosis. *Brit. J. Derm.*, **80**:730, 1968.
119. Shetlar, M. R.: Hypertrophic scar: Hexosamine containing components of burn scars. *Proc. Soc. Exp. Biol. Med.* **139**:544, 1972.
120. Silverman, L. F. and Kove, I.: Atypical epidermoid cyst: A case report. *JAPA*, **49**:641-642, 1959.
121. Skeer, J.: Adenoma sebaceum (Pringle), von Recklinghausen's disease, subungual fibromatosis associated with epilepsy or tuberous sclerosis — a symptom complex. *Urol. Cutan. Rev.*, **42**:110, 1938.
122. Smedal, et al: Ten-year experience with low megavolt electron therapy. *Amer. J. Roentgol.*, **88**:215, 1962.
123. Spencer, D.: Histiocytoma presenting as swelling on the toe. *Arch. Dis. Child.*, **47**:828, 1972.
124. *Stedmans Medical Dictionary.* Williams and Wilkens Company, Baltimore, Maryland, 1966.

125. Stout, A., et al: *Tumors of the Soft Tissues.* Armed Forces Institute of Pathology, Wash., D.C., 1967.
126. Stout, A. P.: Juvenile fibromatosis. *Cancer,* **7**:953-978, 1954.
127. Strahan, R. W., et al: Current concepts in the management of keloids. *Otolaryngol. Clin. N. Amer.,* **5**:521, 1972.
128. Sturim, H. S.: Keloids versus hypertrophic scars. *Rhode Island Medical Journal,* **51**:103, 1968.
130. Tanenbaum, M. H.: Eccrine poroma. *Amer. Surg.,* **31**:603-604, 1965.
131. Tannebaum, N., et al: Scarring from corticosteroid therapy. *Arch. Derm.,* **89**:560, 1964.
132. Taub, J. and Steinberg, M.: Porokeratosis plantaris discreta, a previously unrecognized dermatopathological entity. *Int. J. Derm.,* **9**:83, 1970.
133. Toub, A. H.: Inclusion cyst of the right heel: A case report. *JAPA,* **49**:414, 1959.
134. Trussler, H., et al: Keloids and Hypertrophic Scars. *Arch. Surg.,* **57**:539, 1948.
135. Valles, J.: Intralesional injection of keloids and hypertrophic scars with dermo jet. *Plast. Reconstr. Surg.,* **38**:202, 1966.
136. Van Den Brenk, H., et al: Radiation in the management of keloids and hypertrophic scars. *Brit. J. Surg.,* **47**:595, 1960.
137. Verallo, V. V.: Acquired digital fibrokeratomas. *Br. J. Derm.,* **80**:730-736, 1968.
138. Waddell, G. F.: A hemangioma involving tendons. *J. Bone & Joint Surg.,* **49B**:138, 1967.
139. Warvi, W. N. and Gates, O.: Epithelial cysts and cystic tumors of the skin. *Am. J. Path.,* **19**:765, 1943.
140. Weaver, R. G.: The action of fluocinoline acetonide upon scar tissue formation. *J. Urol.,* **104**:591, 1970.
141. Weinstein, F.: *Principles and Practice of Podiatry.* Lea & Febiger, Phila., 1968, p. 39.
142. Weisfeld, M.: Understanding porokeratosis plantaris discreta. *JAPA,* **63**:138-144, 1973.
143. Wien, M. S. and Caro, M. R.: Traumatic epithelial cysts of the skin. *JAPA,* **102**:197, 1934.
144. Wilson, W.: Prophylaxis against postsurgical keloids. *Southern Med. J.,* **58**:751, 1965.
145. Wright, E., et al: Keloids and ultrasound. *Arch. Phys. Med. Rehab.,* **52**:286, 1971.
146. Wrong, N.: Postoperative Keloids — Treat Or Ignore. *Canad. Med. Assoc. J.,* **101**:226, 1969.
147. Yale, J. F.: Cutaneous mucus cysts of the toes. *JAPA,* 57:457-464, 1967.
148. Yasuda, T., et al: Eccrine proma: A case showing melanin granules and melanocytes in the tumor. *Arch. Derm.,* **90**:428-431, 1964.

Index

A

Acanthosis Nigricans
    Clinical picture, 90
    Definition, 90
    Histopathology, 24
    History, 90
    Onset, 90
    Treatment, 91
    Types, 91
Acne Vulgaris, 188
Actinic Keratosis
    Definition, 82
    Onset, 83
    Treatment, 84
Adenoma Sebaceum, 198
Adnexal Tumors, 148, 181
    Eccrine glands, 181
    Epidermis, 181
    Sebaceous glands, 181
Amelanotic Melanoma, 25, 148, 172
Aneurysms, 135
Alopecia, 111
Angiokeratoma, 73, 93
    Differential diagnosis, 135
Arsenical Keratosis
    Clinical picture, 79
    Differential diagnosis, 64, 80, 156, 172
    Definition, 79
    History, 79
    Onset, 79
    Treatment, 81
Arthritis
    Gonococcal, 110
    Gouty, 92
    Osteo, 94
    Psoriatic, 107
    Rheumatoid, 95
Atrophy, 10
A Vitaminosis, 226

B

Basal Cell Carcinoma, 9, 144
    Clinical picture, 146
    Common errors, 153
    Diagnosis, 147
    Differential, 49, 86, 135, 147, 159, 168, 171, 182
    Etiology, 127, 144
    Fibroepithelioma, 147
    Histopathology, 145
    Introduction, 144
    Natural history, 147
    Pedal involvement, 148
    Nodulo-ulcerative, 135, 145
    Pigmented, 145
    Prognosis, 154
    Rodent, 135, 145
    Sclerosing, 145
    Sites of predilection, 146
    Superficial, 146, 171
    Treatment, 153
Basalioma Cell, 145
Basosquamous Cell Acanthoma, 25
Biopsy, 7
Black Heel, 26, 29
Blisters, 135
Bowen's Disease
    Clinical picture, 169
    Differential diagnosis, 80, 84, 171
    Etiology, 167
    Histological appearance, 169
    Incidence on the pedal extremity, 170
    Introduction, 167
    Relationship to internal cancer, 168
    Treatment, 172
Bullous Pemphigoid, 96
    Differential diagnosis, 97
    Etiology, 97
    Treatment, 97

C

Carcinoma
    Basel cell, 144-154
    Squamous cell, 155-166
    Subungual, 137
Chemotherapy, 11, 33, 39, 51, 54, 67, 70, 76, 81, 84, 94, 96, 98, 104, 106, 110, 141, 153, 172, 214, 218, 221, 226, 228

Chicken Pox (Varicella Virus), 52
Condyloma Acuminata, 36
Contact Dermatitis, 53
Creeping Eruptions, 108, 109
Cryotherapy, 11, 31, 49, 81, 110, 164, 172, 226
Cutaneous Horn
 Clinical picture, 86
 Definition, 85
 Differential, 64
 Histological picture, 87
 Onset, 85
 Treatment, 87
Cutaneous Lava Migrans, 108, 109
Cutaneous Mucous Cysts (Myxoid Cysts)
 Clinical considerations, 219
 Differential diagnosis, 221
 Histopathology, 221
 Literature review, 219
 Prognosis, 221
 Treatment, 221
Cysts, 2, 9

D

Dark Hemangioma, 135
Dermatitis
 Eczematoid, 82
Dermatitis Herpetiformis, 97
Dermatofibroma (Histiocytoma, Sclerosing Hemangioma), 201
 Differential diagnosis, 120, 135, 148, 203
 Histology, 205
Dermatofibrosarcoma Protuberans
 Clinical picture, 222
 Definition, 221
 Differential diagnosis, 205
 Etiology, 222
 Histology, 222
 Incidence, 222
Diabetes Mellitus, 8, 97
 Complications, 100
 Differential diagnosis, 99
 Etiology, 98
 Treatment, 98
Digital Fibrokeratoma, 198
Dyskeratosis Congenita, 92

E

Eccrine Hydrocystoma, 184
Eccrine Mixed Tumor, 184
Eccrine Poroma, 151, 181
 Description, 181
 Differential diagnosis, 25, 48, 182, 184
 Etiology, 181
  Eccrine sweat duct, 182
 Histopathology, 182
 Prognosis, 183
 Treatment, 184
Eccrine Spiradenoma, 184
Eczema Herpeticum, 50
Electrocautery, 12, 36, 67, 81, 84, 87, 141, 153, 164, 172, 228
Elephantiasis Nostras Verrucosa, 93
Epidermal Inclusion Cyst, 9, 188
 Clinical considerations, 190
 Differential diagnosis, 25, 135, 188, 203, 221
 Histology, 221
 Introduction, 188
 Literature review, 190
Epidermoid Carcinoma, 155, 168
Epidermolysis Bullosa, 96
 Differential diagnosis, 97
Epithelioma, 144
Erysipelas, 93
Erythema Elevatum Diutinum
 Clinical picture, 102
 Etiology, 100
 Symptoms, 102
 Treatment, 103
Erythema Multiforme, 97
Excoriations, 2, 10

F

Fatal Black Tumor, 127
Fibroepithelial Papillomas, 25
Fibroma Durum, 195
Fibroma (Inoma), 195, 210
 Angiofibroma, 135
 Clinical picture, 195
 Histopathology, 195, 211
 Introduction, 195
 Prognosis, 195
 Subungual, 137
 Treatment, 196
Fibroma Molle, 195
Fibromatosis
 Dermal, 200
Fibrosarcoma, 203, 221
Fibrous Tumors, 195
Fissures, 10
Fixed Drug Eruption, 97

Differential diagnosis, 137
Follicular Keratosis, 75
Foreign Body Granuloma, 25, 48

G

Ganglionic Cyst, 221
Gangrene, 135
Differential diagnosis, 137
Glomus Tumor, 137, 172
Giant Cell Tumor, 135
Gonococcal Arthritis, 110
Gouty Arthritis, 92
Differential diagnosis, 110
Treatment, 94
Granuloma, 203
Foreign body, 25, 48
Granuloma Annulare
Treatment, 99
Granuloma Fungoides, 104

H

Hand, Foot and Mouth Disease, 53
Hemangioma
Capillary, 203,224, 228
Cavernous, 148
Clinical picture, 225
Diagnosis, 226
Differential diagnosis, 135, 182, 226
Introduction, 223
Prognosis, 228
Spider, 224, 228
Strawberry, 224, 226
Treatment, 226
Hemangio Epithelioma, 135
Hematoma, 25, 131, 137, 208
Herpes Simplex, 9, 50
Clinical picture, 50
Differential diagnosis, 51, 53
Etiology, 50
Treatment, 51
Herpes Zoster (Shingles), 9, 52
Clinical picture, 52
Complications, 53
Differential diagnosis, 53
Etiology, 52
Laboratory diagnosis, 53
Signs and symptoms, 52
Treatment, 54
Hodgkins Disease, 105
Differential diagnosis, 107
Hutchinson's Melanotic Freckle, 125, 135
Hyperhidrosis, 68, 69
Differential diagnosis, 72, 77, 79
Hyperkeratosis, 63
Differential diagnosis, 25, 135
Helloma, 221
Hyperkeratotic lesions, 65
Subungual, 131, 137
Hyperkeratotic Squamous Papilloma, 26

I

Ichthyosis Hystrix, 75
Infantile Dermal Fibromatosis, 200
Infantile Digital Fibromatosis, 200
Intraepidermal Squamous Cell Carcinoma, 167, 168

J

Juvenile Fibromatosis, 198

K

Kaposis Sarcoma, 182
Differential diagnosis, 135, 137
Keloids and Hypertrophic Scars, 205, 219
Differential diagnosis, 166, 222
Etiology, 45, 148, 156, 208
Histology, 210
Introduction, 205
Radiation, 32
Treatment, 214
Keratoacanthoma, 9, 87
Clinical picture, 88
Definition, 87
Differential diagnosis, 49, 148, 172, 203
History, 87
Onset, 87
Treatment, 89
Keratodermia Bienorrhagica, 111
Keratosis (Pre-cancerous), 79
Keratosis Follicularis, 73
Focal, 25
Keratosis Palmaris Et Plantaris Hereditaria (KPPH), 68, 71
Clinical picture, 68
Definition, 68
Differential diagnosis, 168
History, 68

Onset, 68
Treatment, 70
Keratosis Punctata
Clinical picture, 72
Definition, 72
Differential diagnosis, 73
History, 70
Onset, 72
Treatment, 73
Keratosis Striata
Clinical picture, 75
History, 75
Onset, 76
Treatment, 76
Kernan's Tumor, 198
Klippel-Trenaunay Syndrome, 226

L

Lentigo Malignant Melanoma, 125
Leukemia, 105
Lichen Planus, 108
Differential diagnosis, 48, 73
Lichen Simplex, 171
Liver Disease, 226

M

Macules, 2, 9
Mal De Meleda
Clinical picture, 77
Definition, 76
Etiology, 76
History, 76
Onset, 76
Treatment, 77
Malignant Cutaneous Epithelioma, 83
Malignant Lymphoma, 105, 107, 114
Malum Perforans, 81
Differential diagnosis, 100
Marjolin's Ulcer, 157
Mastocytosis Syndrome, 103
Etiology, 104
Treatment, 104
Melanocarcinoma, 125
Melanoma, 119, 121, 125
Age distribution, 132
Differential diagnosis, 123, 134, 148, 182, 203
Digital melanoma, 139
Etiology, 127
Histology, 137
History, 126
Incidence, 141
Introduction, 125
Lentigo maligna, 125, 132
Life cycle, 129
Prepubertal melanoma (juvenile), 131, 135
Prognosis, 145
Regional ratio, 132
Size and symptoms, 130
Subungual melanoma (melanotic whitlow) 131, 135, 136, 139
Treatment, 138
Melanosarcoma, 125
Metastatic Carcimona, 148, 162
Mole, 120
Molluscum Contagiosum, 9, 47
Differential diagnosis, 24, 25, 48
Etiology, 14, 47
Histology, 24, 48
Literature review, 48
Onset, 47
Treatment, 49
Morton's Syndrome, 65
Mycobacterial Infections
Treatment, 104
Types, 104
Mycosis Fungoides, 104
Clinical picture, 106
Differential diagnosis, 106, 107
Treatment, 106
Myrmecia, 20

N

Necrobiosi Lipoidica Diabeticorum, 9, 99
Differential diagnosis, 98
Treatment, 99
Nevi
Benign pigmented, 135
Blue nevus, 119, 121, 122, 135
Compound, 119, 121, 122, 127
Differential diagnosis, 75, 148, 182
Epithelial, 25
Intradermal, 120
Introduction, 119
Junctional, 120, 121, 127
Juvenile melanoma, 119, 123, 132
Life cycle, 124
Mongolian spots, 119, 123

Nevus Graneus, 224
Nevus Flammeus, 224
Nevus Unius Lateris, 75
Nevus Vasculosis, 224
Nodular Hidrodenomes, 25
Nodular Melanoma, 125
Nodules, 2, 9

O

Occupational Keratosis
- Clinical picture, 81
- Definition, 81
- Differential diagnosis, 64
- Onset, 81
- Treatment, 82

Orychomycosis, 137, 172
Osteoarthritis
- Diagnosis, 94
- Heberden's nodes, 94, 221
- Signs and symptoms, 94
- Treatment, 94

Pachyonychia Congenita, 75
Paget's Disease, 135
Papillon - LeFevre Syndrome
- Clinical picture, 77
- History, 77
- Onset, 77
- Treatment, 78

Papules, 9
Paronychia, 131, 158
Panasitic Infections, 108
- Clinical picture, 109
- Treatment, 109

Pemphigus Vulgaris, 51, 96
- Differential diagnosis, 97

Periodontoclasia, 77
Periungual Fibroma
- Clinical picture, 198
- Differential diagnosis, 198
- Etiology, 196
- Histopathology, 198
- Introduction, 196
- Literature review, 196
- Treatment, 198

Pilar Cyst, 8
- Differential diagnosis, 85, 148, 186
- Wen, 187

Piloinidal Cyst, 190
Plaques, 2, 9
Porokeratosis Plantaris Discreta
- Clinical considerations, 24, 184
- Differential diagnosis, 25, 186
- Etiology, 184
- Histopathology, 24, 186
- Incidence, 184
- Introduction, 184

Porokeratosis of Mibelli, 73, 184
- Differential diagnosis, 25

Portwine Stain, 224, 226, 228
Prickle Cell Carcinoma, 155
Prognosis, 12
Psoriasis
- Arthritis, 107
- Differential diagnosis, 73, 148, 171

Pustules, 9
Psychotherapy, 30
Pyogenic Granuloma, 182
- Differential diagnosis, 135, 137, 148, 172, 203

R

Radiation, 12, 30, 81, 99, 106, 172, 214, 221, 226, 228
Recurrent Digital Fibroma of Childhood
- Clinical appearance, 203
- Histology, 205
- Introduction, 200
- Treatment, 205

Reiter's Syndrome
- Clinical picture, 110
- Differential diagnosis, 110
- Etiology, 110
- Treatment, 110

Rendu Osler Weber's Disease, 227
Rheumatoid Arthritis
- Clinical picture, 95
- Differential diagnosis, 99, 110
- Pannus, 95
- R.A. nodule, 95, 96
- Treatment, 96

Sarcoidosis, 103
Sarcoma, 200
Scleroderma, 10, 207
Sclerosis, 10
Sebaneous Cyst (Wen), 8, 178
- Differential diagnosis, 85, 148, 186

Seborrheic Keratosis, 182
- Differential diagnosis, 135, 148

Senile Keratosis, 82

Differential diagnosis, 64, 159, 171
Shingles, 9, 52
Shope Fibroma Virus, 200
Skin
Introduction, 3
Diagnosis, 5
Function, 4
Laboratory diagnosis, 7
Layers, 3
Solar Keratosis, 82, 171
Squamous Cell Carcinoma
Introduction, 155
Etiology, 156
Classification based on source, 157
Clinical picture, 157
Diagnosis, 158
Differential diagnosis, 79, 84, 86, 87, 88, 135, 148, 159, 172, 182
Histopathology, 160
Bone involvement, 160
Matastasis, 162
Distribution, 163
Treatment, 163
Prognosis, 166
Rodent carcinoma, 135
Squamous Cell Carcinoma *in situ*, 167, 169
Stratum Spinosum, 20
Sturge Weber Syndrome, 226
Surgery, 12, 41, 49, 96, 99, 104, 138, 153, 164, 172, 214, 218, 221, 228
Synovial Cyst, 203
Syphilis, 8, 111
Differential diagnosis, 73, 80, 103
Tabes dorsalis, 112
Syringoma, 184

T

Tinea Nigra, 135
Tinea Pedis, 53
Treatment, 11
Trichinosis, 103
Tuberculosis, 103
Type, 104
Tuberous Sclerosis, 8, 196
Differential diagnosis, 25, 198

U

Ulcers, 2, 10
Ultrasound, 214
Unna-Thost Disease, 68
Differential diagnosis, 77
Urticaria Pigmentosa, 104

V

Varicella (Chickenpox) Virus, 52
Varices, 135
Vasculitis, 103
Necrotizing, 102
Verruca Plantaris
Clinical consideration, 23
Complications, 45
Condyloma acuminata (moist wart), 36
Differential diagnosis, 24, 48, 73, 86, 87, 135, 148, 182, 186, 198
Etiology, 18
Histopathology, 24
Incidence, 18, 21
Mosaic verruca, 17, 19, 33, 34
Papova virus, 17
Pathogenesis, 19
Prognosis, 45
Subungual verruca, 21, 33, 35
Treatment, 28
Verruca Vulgaris, 17, 48, 221
Vesicles and Bullae, 9, 221
Viral Tumors
Introduction, 3, 17
Vitamin B Deficiency, 226
Von Recklinghausen's Disease, 8, 198
Differential diagnosis, 135, 200
Xanthoma Diabeticorum, 99, 101
Differential diagnosis, 221
Treatment, 100